INTERPRETING
CHRONIC
ILLNESS

"Jerry Kantor has successfully integrated the disciplines of homeopathy, acupuncture, and biomedicine into pragmatic healing approaches that busy practitioners can readily and easily apply to common clinical presentations. Multimodal management and integrative medicine techniques, while certainly the best approach to medical conditions, can be deceptively complex. Jerry's explanations and guidelines are the perfect balance of background information and recommendations, allowing the clinician to effectively supplement their treatment armamentarium."

—Mark Scheutzow, MD, PhD, DHom, NMD
FAAIM, DABHM, DAAPM

"A brilliant and groundbreaking work by an integrative practitioner who 'speaks the language' of three very different healing paradigms—biomedicine (modern Western medicine), Traditional Chinese Medicine and homeopathy. By illuminating each in the light of the others, he brings the CAM [complementary and alternative medicine] modalities from a subservient role as 'alternative medicine' to full participation as 'complementary.' Kantor simultaneously updates the Five Elements model of Traditional Chinese Medicine; provides fresh insights into the major homeopathic remedies based on the Five Elements model; and shows how both can address the diagnostic categories of biomedicine. This will be an essential book for practitioners and students of all three modalities who want to expand their healing paradigm."

—Begabati Lennihan, RN, CCH
Former Director
Teleosis School of Homeopathy

"A seminal work of probing, integrative intelligence, Jerry Kantor's book *Interpreting Chronic Illness* systematically lays out how Nature, personal temperament and life experience constitute the crucible for chronic illness and, in turn, the laboratory for self-understanding. It will consolidate and advance the thinking of practitioners of acupuncture and homeopathy, and will challenge Western-trained health care professionals to think of illness and disease as more than just invading pathogens."

> —Eugene L. Pogany, PhD, Clinical Psychologist
> Author
> *In My Brother's Image*

"Much of American medicine is based on the belief that disease is an entity that flies through the air and lands on the unlucky, whereupon we 'do battle' with it. Jerry Kantor persuades us otherwise with his thoroughly original coalescence of the best of Eastern and Western views of diagnosis and treatment. I won't let another physician touch me until he/she has read this book."

> —William Martin Sloane, PhD
> Vice President
> American Association of Integrative Medicine

"I know of no other body of work, in the science of homeopathic medicine, which demystifies the core essence of homeopathic materia medica as does Kantor's brilliant work. A truly integrative, evidence-based perspective that should be mandatory reading for all practitioners of the art, science and philosophy of homeopathy."

> —Georgianna Donadio, PhD
> Florence Nightingale Scholar
> Director
> National Institute of Whole Health

"This is an excellent book for those of us who would like to use both Traditional Chinese Medicine, including acupuncture and homeopathy, to treat patients."

—Zhaoming Chen, MD, PhD, MS, CFP, FAAIM, LAc
Chair and Chief Spokesman
American Association of Integrative Medicine
Diplomate of Neurology and Clinical Neurophysiology
American Board of Psychiatry and Neurology
Certified Qigong Instructor
Tai Chi Master

"Jerry Kantor has produced a book that is wise, perceptive, practical and immediately applicable, but that will also yield further riches on deep study. It draws on the three apparently incompatible fields of acupuncture, homeopathy and modern biomedicine, and weaves from them whole cloth: a patterned approach to understanding chronic illness, and guidelines for treatment. Worthy of serious consideration."

—Steven Clavey, Dip Adv Acupuncture
Author
Fluid Physiology and Pathology in Chinese Medicine

"This book is a major triangulation of multi-medical perspectives that add to our understanding of what healing is about. Jerry Kantor has done a great job!"

—Ted Kaptchuk, OMD
Author
The Web That Has No Weaver:
Understanding Chinese Medicine

INTERPRETING
CHRONIC
ILLNESS

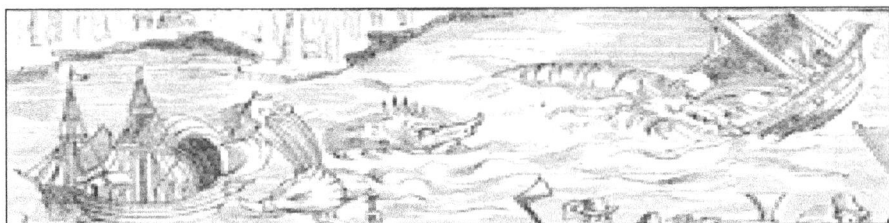

INTERPRETING CHRONIC ILLNESS

THE CONVERGENCE OF TRADITIONAL CHINESE MEDICINE HOMEOPATHY AND BIOMEDICINE

JERRY M. KANTOR
LIC AC, CCH, MMHS

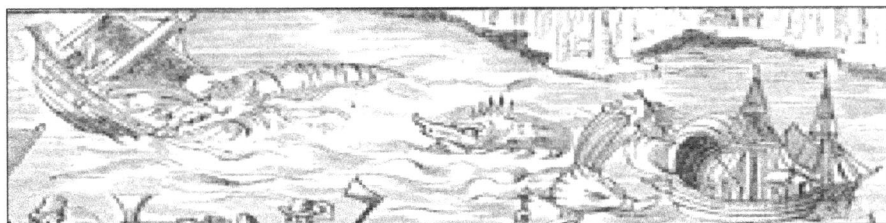

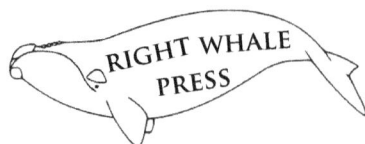

RIGHT WHALE
PRESS

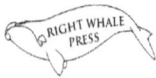

RIGHT WHALE PRESS
332 Washington Street, Suite 280
Wellesley Hills, MA 02481

For permission requests, write to the publisher, addressed as follows: Attention: Permissions Coordinator, Right Whale Press, 332 Washington Street, Suite 280, Wellesley Hills, MA 02481. Web site: www.Rightwhalepress.com.

The material in this book is not meant to take the place of diagnosis and treatment by a medical doctor or a licensed therapist.

Ordering Information:
Quantity sales: Special discounts are available on quantity purchases by corporations, associations, and others. For details, contact Right Whale Press at the address above.

Orders by U.S. trade bookstores and wholesalers: Contact CreateSpace at www.createspace.com, and sign up as a reseller with CreateSpace Direct.

Book and cover designed by Doris Yokelson

Printed in the United States of America

Publisher's Cataloging-in-Publication Data
Kantor, Jerry.
Chronic illness: the convergence of traditional Chinese medicine, homeopathy, and biomedicine / Jerry Kantor — 1st ed.
p.   cm.
Includes bibliographical references and index.
1. Medicine—Homeopathy—Traditional Chinese Medicine—Psychology.
2. Phenomenology.   3. Chronic illness from Integrative Medicine perspective.
I. Title.
Library of Congress Control Number: 2011917625
First Edition: December 2011
ISBN 978-0-9846788-0-8

FOR HANNAH

From youth we are seafarers
hoping to attain the distant
shore of healthful old age.
Success requires our navigating
a perilous strait; for we must
manage to sail past the Scylla
of cancer on one side and
the Charybdis of chronic
illness on the other.

Medicine and sickness cure one
another. The whole earth is
medicine. Where do you find
the self?
—Master Unmon

All ensouled bodies are the
drops of the Ocean of all
Consciousness. When we know
this, all is beautiful.
—Master Kirpal Singh

ACKNOWLEDGMENTS

Thanks go out to the late Dr. James Tin Yao So who initiated me into the healing arts. I am also grateful to David Kailin, Robert Weissberg, MD, and Leonard Goldberg for their valuable input in the preparation of this manuscript. Any and all errors contained herein are mine alone!

Others to whom I am grateful for the varieties of their support are Karen Allen, Georgianna Donadio, Claudia Kalberg, Begabati Lennihan, Ken Lubowich, Wendy Marks, Patricia Purcell, Sally Lueth, and Lyn Swirda.

It is to the nonpareil Doris Yokelson, inspired graphic artist and consummate editor and researcher embedded within my own family, that I owe the bulk of my gratitude. Thank you, Doris, for your elegant rendering of my ideas!

I also wish to express loving appreciation and gratitude to my wife Hannah and my daughter Zoe for seeing me so patiently through this project.

Not least, I wish to thank my many patients who lived the ideas conveyed in this book at close range, and for whom the experience of illness came to signify exploration.

CONTENTS

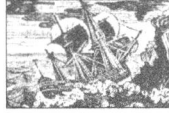
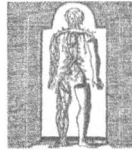
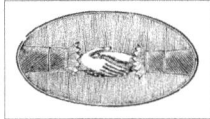

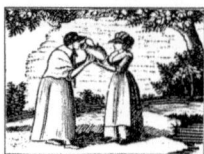

CHAPTER FOUR
The Dimension of Taste

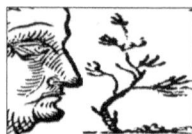

CHAPTER FIVE
The Dimension of Smell

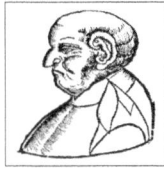

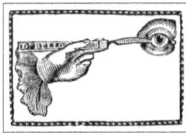

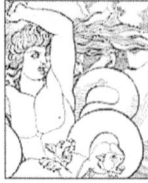

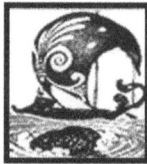

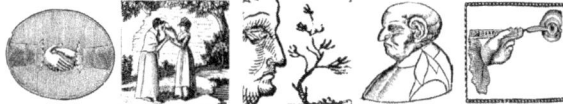

CHAPTER TEN

CREATE YOUR OWN FIVE SENSE DIMENSIONAL MANDALA

EPILOGUE: TURNING OUR GREAT SHIP

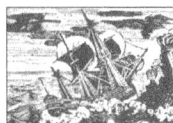

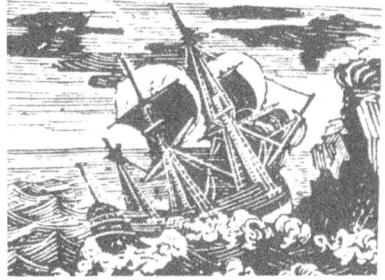

CHAPTER ONE

TURNING OUR GREAT SHIP: A SEA CHANGE

Our Great Ship—our human form—is built of dreams, physical and emotional needs, and unique capabilities, fashioned to withstand life's squalls, gales, and treacherous currents. The Sea of Life on which our Great Ship sails has also been given to us as a source of primal life energy.

A ship at sea and the wide sea maintain a tenuous relationship. A ship is buoyed, and the sea yields up its bountiful life for the sailors; yet often trade winds and perfect storms buffet the ship and destroy it. Like a ship at sea, our Great Ship endures life's volatility and discovers that the Sea of Life is neither unlimited nor unconditionally ours.

In this book I offer a new model to redirect our Great Ship, measure for measure, toward the health-giving, primal energy of the Sea of Life.

PHENOMENOLOGY: THE GREAT SHIP'S WHEEL

Phenomenology's model of nondualistic phenomenon provides the ideological framework for converging the principles and practices of Eastern and Western aspects of medicine—in other words, for constructing a new model of interpreting chronic illness and for steering our Great Ship, degree by degree, toward the primal energy of the Sea of Life.

In philosophy, phenomenology is broadly defined as a theoretical approach toward understanding how people experience the world they live in and create.

1

Phenomenology was posited by the early twentieth century philosopher Edmund Husserl as a method of analyzing human existence and state of being without making prior assumptions—in other words, studying, without presuppositions, the nature of human experience and consciousness in everyday life.

Can we possibly observe and analyze human life without starting from presuppositions or prior assumptions? Can we also possibly observe and analyze chronic illness in the same way—that is, as an entirety, as a unity of phenomena, without any presuppositions or assumptions derived from evidence-based perspectives? A patient's chronic illness is conveyed to us through the phenomenon of his or her narrative, an unformatted mountain of data not limited to its spoken elements. Before a course of treatment can be decided, the essential meaning encrypted within the text of the patient's illness must be decoded. How is this even possible? Where are we to begin?

To approach answering this at all, we have to develop a new model for the understanding and healing of chronic illness, a model built on the observation and awareness of the unity and integrity of the natural phenomena of illness. The system introduced in this book—even with its openness to empirical testing—originates in an intuitively-based means of analysis, which, in turn, is grounded in the concept of phenomenology.

Phenomenology can be applied to many different fields; its precepts extend beyond philosophy to infuse disciplines as diverse as ecology, anthropology, history, literary criticism, sociology, ethnology, psychology, and medicine. For the purpose here of examining chronic illness, phenomenology's key relevant features provide us with the following excellent tools for an in-depth analysis.

A focus on genuine life issues.

Phenomenology asserts experiential immediacy, that is, the primacy of the five senses in detecting, shaping, and fusing the mental constructs of the world around us. The senses function by merging a person's external world of stimuli with that of his or her internal consciousness. A key thesis of this book is that each of the five senses, in fact, constitutes in itself an entire separate dimension of distinctive traits.

A means by which we can understand how the unity of a phenomenon prefigures knowledge of its components.

We need a method to describe a universal *something*, an *a priori* structure underlying cognition, with which we can shape our sense of causality and provide objects within their context. Subjective intention generally shapes our perception of most objects. As Abraham Maslow[1] says, "If the only tool you have is a hammer you tend to see every problem as a nail." How are we to break through this wall of subjective intention which inevitably shapes our perception?

Phenomenology offers a way to do this, a method known as phenomenological, or eidetic, reduction. This method involves identifying and then removing hindrances to a clearer and more definite understanding of something, thus eliminating irrelevancies and culture-bound influences. As the grounding of a given phenomenon starts to take shape, its essential meaning begins to emerge. In the practitioner's study of chronic illness, the failure to recognize the impact of one's own subjective intention or role—as in transference reactions or self-investment in a particular outcome—may undermine the effectiveness of treatment.

A basis for common-sense perceptions of mind-body unity.

During the Enlightenment, the idea that the mind and the body exist in separate spheres was cogently expressed by the great French mathematician and philosopher René Descartes. Phenomenology grew out of the recognition that this dualistic perspective inadequately describes the richness of lived experience.

Without this lived, unifying richness, everything seemingly accomplished appears to be a chimera. Ralph Waldo Emerson noted something analogous to this about writers in his personal journal:

> Chaucer, Milton and Shakespeare have seen mountains, if they speak of them. The young writers seem to have seen pictures of mountains. The wish to write poetry they have, but not the poetic fury; and what they write is studies, sketches, fantasies, and not yet the inestimable poem.[2]

TURNING OUR GREAT SHIP: A SEA CHANGE

Each of us enters the world with specific physical traits, temperaments, mental gifts, and quirks. No one of us is a blank slate, a *tabula rasa*. Unique and inherent characteristics, such as our ease or difficulty in adjusting to an unfamiliar situation, strongly influence the strength or weakness of our constitution, the chief determinant of our susceptibility to illness. It is good to keep in mind that by "susceptibility" the *potential* for illness and not the *guarantee* of illness is meant. Susceptibility to an illness need not progress to the level of disease.

Illnesses are often kaleidoscopic. The spectrum of an individual's expression of disease rivals that of personality or of intelligence. Although many causes may be presumed for a disease, each is, in reality, only a potential cause of disease. Whether an actual pathogen develops, and the degree to which it manifests, is a reflection of an individual's constitution, a strong one obviously being more resilient and a delicate one more sensitive to the potential causes. Further, a focus on the symptoms of disease obscures the genuine importance of life-history issues that underlie the disease process. The good news is that, under favorable conditions, the body can have the capacity to reverse the process of many illnesses regarded today as merely manageable or as simply hopeless.

A Spyglass

Professional training in effect provides the health care practitioner with a spyglass on the world. It has been my personal good fortune to have received three spyglasses and a directive to map a unifying perspective. The three—none of which alone provides a total picture of illness—are homeopathy, Traditional Chinese Medicine, and biomedicine. Of these, Traditional Chinese Medicine and its theoretical system, reconfigured around the five senses, provides the framework of the book's organizing superstructure and its novel model of chronic illness.

As will be shown, each of the senses represents not only a body of knowledge that codes our *a priori* connection to nature, but a dimension, the resolution of whose core issue promotes health and development. Our ability to map—that is, to organize symptoms according to sense-dimensional themes—prompts the directive nestled within an illness to come to light, and a partnering strategy for the reversal of the illness to be crafted.

A View From the Wheelhouse

Master Unmon, born in Jiaxing, China, in 864, was a renowned Zen teacher within a Taoist-influenced Buddhist school of thought known as Chán. The Master one day asked his students this question:

> Medicine and sickness cure one another. The whole earth is medicine. Where do you find the self?[3]

Master Unmon had presented here a *koan* (in Zen, "riddle"). In order for his students to extract and gain possession of wisdom to be found inside the *koan*, they had to grapple with the answer on their own. I will share my own answer, after first rephrasing Master Unmon's question:

> It is easy to see that medicine can cure sickness, but how can sickness cure medicine? What does medicine need to be cured of? Sickness can cure medicine when treatment shortcomings and failures are acknowledged, new perspectives are sought, and the course of therapeutic actions are thereby altered.

In seeking where you find the self, Master Unmon referred to the Buddhist doctrine of the insubstantiality of identity. Yet the context suggests something more here: The specifics of an individual's immediate situation are crucial to health, sickness, and cure; the selection of correct interventions rests upon profound comprehension and respect for these specifics and for the person.

To say that the whole earth is medicine is to acknowledge the interlinkage of all creation. As cause and cure are multifactorial, health and diseases do not arise independently. Master Unmon reminds us of the need for flexibility in our perspectives, as well as the need for acumen in our selection of therapeutic measures.

What is it that will ultimately prove therapeutic for chronic illness? A hoped-for apology, the puncture of a fine needle, a retribution, the reading or writing of a poem, a vivid dream, the surgeon's steel, the pulling of weeds from a garden, the infusions of a course herb, a drum beat, snake venom diluted many hundredfold . . . each has its moment of curative power.

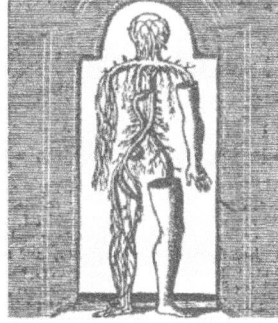

CHAPTER TWO

BEYOND BIOMEDICINE

Possession of a map greatly aids the Great Ship's voyage of discovery. The map we unfold throughout this book conveys the basis for our perspectives on the territory of chronic illness. The brief explanations we offer provide only the rudiments of the map. Medical professionals will recognize the need for deeper study to master the concepts addressed. Yet nonmedical readers will grasp the essential ideas that orient the voyage.

Chronic illnesses would be less prevalent and less devastating if we could fully understand their causes and effectively apply that understanding. To some extent, prevailing biomedical understandings of chronic illness are incomplete. That leads us to consider chronic illnesses from the additional perspectives of Traditional Chinese Medicine (TCM) and homeopathy.

Each theoretical approach and each model of a situation acts like a lens. A lens has a focal point of clarity, areas of distortion, and blind spots (absolute limits). By bringing the three lenses of biomedicine, TCM, and homeopathy to bear conjointly on the problem of chronic illness, we can apply their combined power to produce a more telling map. As we shall come to see, lenses sometimes need a little polishing to perform their best.

The lens of biomedicine is well-developed and powerful. Although biomedical perspectives are cited throughout this book, a full account of what biomedicine has provided in the way of genetic, biochemical, and biological insights cannot be provided. That portion of the map is already detailed elsewhere and extensive.

BUILDING THE FRAMEWORK

Traditional Chinese Medicine (TCM)

TCM's contributions to medicine are extensive, stemming from the historical depth of its clinical and theoretical development. But its contributions are not well appreciated in the West, obscured as TCM is across a vast cultural divide. Assuming different premises, TCM holds remarkably dissimilar conceptions from Western biomedicine of the body and of the nature and functions of its organs. Throughout this book, when we refer to an organ as conceived of in TCM, we will capitalize the organ name—for example, Heart—to distinguish it from the organ as conceived of in biomedicine—heart. An admirable introduction to TCM is *The Web That Has No Weaver: Understanding Chinese Medicine,* by Ted Kaptchuk.[1]

TCM depicts the transformation of environmental energy and substances into energy, termed Qi, and substances of the body. This process is dynamic, cyclical, and multileveled. Within the body, the organs circulate Qi, blood, and other fluids. They act together in relationship, nourishing, harnessing, and balancing each other. Illnesses in TCM originate from specific environmental exposures, excesses, deficiencies, stagnations, and misdirections of the flow of energy. Health represents a balance of opposing yet complementary forces, expressed in terms of Yin and Yang (see **Table 1**).

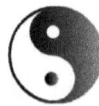

Table 1. Attributes of Yin and Yang

YIN	feminine	receptive	cool	dark	moist	earth	matter
YANG	masculine	active	hot	bright	dry	heaven	energy

TCM posits an integral connectivity between an organism and the environment and between the organs and the organism. These relationships are expressed in the Five-Phases, or Five-Elements, theory (see **Figure 1** and **Table 2**). Why five and not four or six Phases? In his book, *The Reflexive Universe,* Arthur Young[2] points out that the minimum number of loci from which a geometric diagram of the storage of energy can be constructed is five. Thus, when the Moebius strip, which contains energy because the twists in the strip store tension, is mapped onto a two-dimensional surface, the result is a pentagon figure, familiar to practitioners of Five-Phase acupuncture.

According to TCM, in health Qi flows clockwise in a Generating Cycle from one Phase into the next succeeding Phase (e.g., from Wood to Fire), generating or promoting the next Phase. Qi also flows clockwise from one Phase into the Phase that is two positions after it (e.g., from Wood to Earth). This controls, harnesses, or supports the recipient Phase and its related organs. Illness can indicate disharmonious Phase conditions or Phase relationships. The Generating Cycle and the relationships between Phases are detailed in Chapter 9; the bodily functions and symptoms associated with each Phase are described in Chapters 3 to 7.

Figure 1. Five-Phases Pentagram

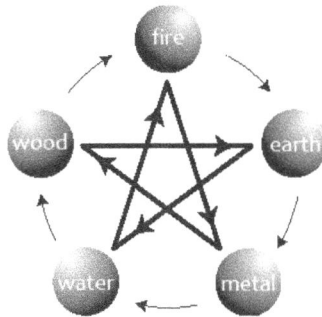

Note in **Table 2** that taste is represented twice and that touch (having no discrete orifice) is conspicuously absent. Strictly speaking, traditional TCM sources associate the Heart with the tongue as its sense organ and then provide no sense dimension. But taste is logically the sense dimension to associate with the tongue. We may realize then that the traditional TCM designations are partially in error and in need of reconsideration. These errors have been passed down through the centuries. Such is the regard for the ancient tradition that no one has had the temerity to correct an obvious series of mistakes.

The association of taste with the Earth Phase is very well-developed. The Earth Phase concerns food, digestion, and metabolism. Taste is clearly the most

Table 2. Attributes of Five-Phases Pentagram

	FIRE	EARTH	METAL	WATER	WOOD
SEASON	Summer	Long summer	Autumn	Winter	Spring
DIRECTION	South	Center	West	North	East
YIN ORGAN	Heart	Spleen	Lung	Kidney	Liver
YANG ORGAN	Small Intestine	Stomach	Large Intestine	Bladder	Gall Bladder
EMOTION	Joy	Pensiveness	Sadness	Fear	Anger
VOCAL QUALITY	Laughing	Singing	Crying	Groaning	Shouting
TASTE	Bitter	Sweet	Pungent	Salty	Sour
SENSE ORGAN	Tongue (?)	Mouth (?)	Nose	Ears	Eyes
SENSE DIMENSION	Taste (?)	Taste	Smell	Hearing	Sight
PATHOLOGY LEVEL	Transient symptoms Neurosis	Acute symptoms	Periodic symptoms	Susceptibility to addictions Inherited diseases	Chronic symptoms
LIFE STAGE	Childhood	Adolescence	Adult	Midlife	Old age/death

appropriate sense dimension to associate with the Earth Phase; therefore, we should question the attribution of taste to the Fire Phase. The mouth is established as the Earth Phase's associated sense organ, although the tongue would be the more accurate association. Here we should question the attribution of the tongue as the sense organ of the Fire Phase and the Heart.

In TCM, the Heart and Mind form an inseparable unity. The tongue is called "the sprout of the Heart," not because of its tasting functions but because of its speaking functions. The wagging tongue gives vent to the Heart/Mind. Furthermore, the tongue offers diagnostically invaluable information by way of its coating, color, and shape. Through a visual diagnosis of the tongue we can assess the heart of the matter. The tongue's associations with the Heart are too important to be ignored, but its Heart-related functions do not include taste.

What is the Heart's associated sense dimension? After probing this question for years, we have come to accept the obvious. Touch, the overlooked sense dimension in TCM, should be associated with the Phase of Fire and the Heart. This relationship is developed in Chapter 3.

If touch is the sense dimension of the Heart, then the skin (and not the tongue) should be the sense organ of the Heart. Yet skin disorders are primarily associated with the Phase of Metal and the Lungs. The association of a sense organ with a visceral organ suggests that disorders of the sense organ may involve the visceral organ. But this implication is neither strict nor exclusive. A pathology of the eye does not always involve a pathology of the Liver, just as a pathology of the skin does not always involve a pathology of the Lung. The skin as a sense organ can logically be attributed to the Heart without altering the standard clinical understandings of skin disorders in TCM.

Finally, if the sense organ of the Heart is the skin, then the sense organ of the Spleen can be adjusted from the mouth to the tongue. This minor alteration has no significant impact on clinical reasoning in TCM. It is the last correction needed on **Table 2** showing the attributes of the Five Phases.

The Concept of Sense Dimensions

We have now established proper associations between various sense dimensions and Phases in TCM. What is the significance of these associations? The issue is not well-developed in TCM. A sense dimension encompasses much more than just a sense organ. The heart of this book is an exploration of chronic illness through the novel concept of sense dimensions, their core issues and disturbances, and their impact on theories of pathology and healing in TCM, biomedicine, and homeopathy.

Each sense confronts specific aspects of the world and internalizes them. Interpenetration of the senses with the outer world grounds human nature in outer nature at every level of existence. A sense dimension is a dynamic interface between inner and external reality, a Kantian manifold. As opposed to a data machine, each sense dimension is suffused with *a priori* information about how to

Table 3. Attributes of the Sense Dimensions and TCM's Five Phases

SENSE DIMENSION	AXIS OF CORE ISSUE	PHASE	YIN ORGAN	FUNCTION
Touch	Synchrony-Isolation	Fire	Heart	Circulatory
Taste	Challenge-Anxiety	Earth	Spleen	Digestive
Smell	Centeredness-Disorientation	Metal	Lung	Respiratory
Hearing	Consolidation-Entropy	Water	Kidney	Reproduction
Sight	Creativity-Chaos	Wood	Liver	Neural

resolve archetypical issues at its core. The embodiment of Schopenhauer's concept of the Will, the sense dimension is intent upon shaping the perceptual universe. This model of sense dimensions is thus fundamentally at odds with the notions of contemporary thinkers such as Daniel Dennett[3] for whom consciousness is an unmeaning matter, a mechanical hum produced by the brain's computer-like processing of undifferentiated sense data.

We do not come to meet the world empty-handed, but arrive with archetypical human concerns already shaped. For example, the taste's distinction between nutrients and toxins (as well as the gnawing edge of hunger itself) figures into our primal anxiety. Our mastery of anxiety provides the foundation for meeting challenges; anxiety and challenge are the poles of an axis of human concerns, the core issues associated with the sense dimension of taste.

Core issues are most easily recognized at the levels of the conscious and subconscious mind. But our fundamental concerns also play out on higher and lower levels than these. The core issue of anxiety is experienced by organs and by cells, as well as within families, communities, and societies. Failure to adequately resolve core issues at any level can lead to manifestations of illness. The origins of chronic illness are not necessarily located in individual conscious and subconscious mental patterns, although these patterns may contribute to both the cause and cure of illness.

By means of phenomenological analysis we can produce a picture of the core issues associated with the five sense dimensions (**Table 3**). With each of the five successive chapters of this book, we will build a larger framework of understanding: each of the five sense dimensions is explained; the chronic-illness pathologies pertaining to each sense dimension are specified and looked at from a biomedical, homeopathic, and TCM viewpoint, as appropriate; a materia medica of homeo-pathic remedies is provided whose essential themes are matched with the specific issues related to each sense dimension; implications for the maintenance of sense-dimensional vibrancy are suggested; and examples are given of persons who have achieved mastery of one of the sense dimension's two opposing poles on the axis of human concerns.

Homeopathy

Having briefly touched on TCM as a basic component of our analysis, we turn next to homeopathy. Homeopathy was developed by Samuel Hahn-emann in the early 19th century. Its central tenet is that there is therapeutic power in minute doses of substances that produce symptoms similar to those the patient is experiencing,

Why might a homeopathic remedy be effective at all? The homeopathic prescription is highly customized to the individual's situation. The homeopathic practitioner considers not only the biomedical symptoms, but also a broad range of behavioral, attitudinal, emotional, and mental characteristics. In this way, a pattern that matches one of the homeopathic remedies may be understood. The practitioner must search for themes from the patient's life, core issues, entrenched conflicts, and standing problems. This close matching suggests that there may be a high degree of sensitivity to the remedy, such that very little is needed to provoke a response. While acupuncture draws on the innate sensitivity of specific acupuncture points, a homeopathic remedy draws on the innate sensitivity of specific substances. Both rely on the body's life energy—Qi, or the vital force—to bring about healing.

Furthermore, between each unique person and her environment multiple levels exist of commonalities, resonances, and homologies. We are shaped by the world, and each of its creations holds and mirrors specific aspects of our own con-dition. A remedy provides a subtle reminder of a lost or blocked essence, a sorely-missed intelligence that is then recognized and disproportionately responded to by the body. Note that acupuncture also achieves disproportionate effects, using the subtle stimuli of hair-thin needles.

A homeopathic remedy seems to act as a minute provocation, challenge, or irritation. The right remedy prompts a resolution of symptoms across a range of characteristics examined; it does so typically after an initial flare-up, aggravation, or full-fledged catharsis. In the aftermath, the patient's situation may have changed sufficiently enough to display a different pattern or remedy state. Occasionally the transformation occurs so smoothly that it passes unnoticed.

The patient may now be encountering a different layer of his disorder, or his condition may have swung to an opposing position of imbalance. Sometimes the patient is markedly resistant to the changes that have occurred. In the treatment of chronic illness, layers of disturbance are lifted, and gradually the symptom swings become less extreme.

The text of a chronic illness may contain annotations from an ancient hand. Here the homeopath notes the presence of a miasmatic layer, the symptoms and susceptibilities of a disease that had afflicted an ancestor at some earlier time. Consolidated in the germ line, these qualities have been transmitted to the patient. In Chapter 6 we will learn how, within the dimension of hearing, activity on behalf of consolidation resists entropy.

The process whereby successive remedy layers are peeled away may be compared to the action of a simple, slow-moving pendulum. In this metaphor, a remedy state represents the far point of the pendulum's arc in one direction. Resolution of the issue underlying the remedy state frees the pendulum's weight to swing in the opposite direction. Rather than come to a full stop at the point of balance, the pendulum's weight swings in the other direction, bypassing the arc's midpoint. In a pendulum swing—not to be confused with a mere switch in polar features common even within one remedy picture (such as opposing tendencies to be cold as well as warm)—a well-indicated second remedy prompts the process to be repeated. The pendulum's weight once again is released and free to swing in the opposite direction, past the midpoint of the arc. But we now notice that loss of kinetic energy shortens the pendulum's arc. The gradual shortening of the pendulum's arc represents movement in the direction of normalization and an improvement in the status of the patient's health. Thus, for example, a not unreasonable treatment goal for a truly bipolar individual would be to transform him into a moody individual.

The aftermath of a remedy state reveals even more specific evidence that a pendulum swing has occurred: key features of the preceding remedy state are not only ameliorated, but reversed. For example, Sulphur is a complement of Calcarea carbonica. Thus, a physically chilly and intellectually cautious Calcarea carbonica individual can morph into an overheated, mentally overstimulated Sulphur individual. A Lycopodium person, too insecure to speak in front of a group, often swings into a complementary Kali carbonicum state in which excessively self-certain opinions are expressed. An overly intellectualized Calcarea sulphurica individual can morph into a highly sentimental person needing Antimonium crudum.

In TCM's Generating Cycle, a generic form of energy, Qi, cycles from one Phase to the next. Because none of us is a generic individual, our passage from one remedy state to another is neither cyclic nor predictable. However, it is evident that each of TCM's Five Phases holds an affinity for specific homeopathic remedies. Because the remedies possess variants of essentially the same Five-Phase core themes, each is rooted in the human condition. This accounts for the prevalence within clinical practice of select remedies that have come to be called polycrests.

The list includes, but is not limited to, Sulphur and Belladonna manifesting Fire; Lycopodium and Graphites manifesting Earth; Silicea and Natrium muriaticum manifesting Metal; Calcarea carbonica, the Lanthanides, and the miasmatic remedies manifesting Water; Sepia, Stramonium, and Rhus toxicodendron manifesting Wood. In accordance with a method that maps their features across a template consisting of all of the Five Phases, these and other remedies will later be analyzed in detail.

The Concept of Radical Disjunct

Another useful approach comes from identifying the key contradictions or paradoxes that are called here "radical disjuncts." Reminiscent of the ego-defense mechanism described by Sigmund Freud as a reaction formation, a radical disjunct occurs when provision of the normal fulfillment of a need not only fails to quench the need but makes it worse.

Consider the situation of a woman who fears being anywhere close to dirt. She then becomes so vigilant concerning cleanliness that in her drive to eradicate filth she finds herself constantly near it. Here, fear of contacting dirt creates more contact with dirt. This self-reinforcing feedback loop then builds on and perpetuates itself. As opposed to the reaction formation, which describes behavior, the radical disjunct's capacity to encompass physical symptomatology sustains an imbalance or a chronic illness. Sense-dimensional analysis generally illuminates the radical disjuncts that are operant in chronic illness.

Identification of the radical disjunct is central to deconstructing complex and often paradoxical descriptions of homeopathic remedies. For example, the radical disjunct of the homeopathic remedy Nux vomica lies in its indication for a situation in which a person is constantly at war with the world in order "to obtain a little peace." Physically, a patient in need of Nux vomica shows, on the one hand, excessive energy, and on the other, exhaustion; they ought logically to cancel one another out, but fail to do so. A radical disjunct can be created iatrogenically, as when a medication for depression generates increased risk for suicide, or a medication to treat softening of the bones and susceptibility to fracture causes the bones to become brittle.

Underlying each radical disjunct is failure at some level to adequately resolve an issue. The failure ultimately implicates one of the core issues related to the five sense dimensions. Sidestepping these issues with inadequate resolutions sets up patterns of dysfunction that ultimately are expressed in chronic illnesses.

Because remedy-state patterns are complex and a broad perspective is needed to understand them, the intent of this book is not primarily clinical. Rather, it introduces an innovative conceptual tool—sense-dimensional analysis—as a means to conjoin prominent though culturally diverse medical systems. Although health caregivers are encouraged to view their patients' illnesses through the lens of the sense dimensions, they are advised not to exceed the limits of their professional training in treating any psycho-social disturbances they may expose. They are particularly urged not to prescribe homeopathic remedies for chronic illnesses without first undergoing a thorough course of homeopathic training.

WHY INTERPRET SYMPTOMS?

Rather than a standard medical diagnosis of a disease, our methodology is an interpretation of the symptoms of a patient's a chronic illness. A medical diagnosis launches a treatment protocol, while an interpretation of symptoms suggests a plan of care that takes into account the complexity and individual nature of the case, which guarantees that it is to be neither easily nor quickly determined.

Health care practitioners are not immune to the impatience of modern society. The pressure to provide a quick fix comes from so many directions: friends, family members, the workplace, insurers, and the patients themselves. Who among practitioners has not at some time capitulated, offering treatment prematurely, realizing only after the case has developed itself more fully in his mind, that the original plan of action was off base? Clearly, rushing to judge the meaning of symptoms is a bad idea, and specific reasons exist as to why a conscientious search for meaning is worth the trouble. The sections below explain why.

Deepening Understanding and Strengthening the Bond With the Patient

Suppose for a moment that I am given a magic wand that is able to cure every patient over whose head I wave it. Unless the wand gives me true insights into the illness I want to cure, I will immediately hand it back to the giver. In order to heal, I must first understand; only by virtue of understanding can I hope to heal. Curiosity, keenness of observation, and acuity of assessment offer multiple results in the clinical setting. Not the least of these is that both sides of the clinician/client relationship at times sparkle with insight, possibility, joy, and hope.

Promoting the Possibility of a Talking-based or Behavioral-based Cure

Whether or not one is a psychotherapist, there can be times when discussing an analysis of the case with the patient will, in and of itself, be curative. In my own practice, because I generally administer a remedy in my office immediately after deciding a case, such an opportunity seldom presents itself. But instances have occurred—for example, when the patient prefers to give himself the remedy at home—in which a pattern of long-standing symptoms somehow resolves itself before the patient takes the remedy. Such improvement can be lasting, requiring recourse neither to a remedy nor to any other kind of intervention.

Case analysis may also suggest that the therapist use a stratagem based on non-insight, a behavioral prescription requiring that the patient deliberately exaggerate the positive pole of the remedy state's radical disjunct. Prior to entering a Sepia state, for example, a woman who is a candidate for this remedy is normally hopeful. Traumatized by resentment and disappointment, the woman is subsequently ensnared in Sepia. She now comes to experience hope as toxic, as a result of which her energy undergoes profound stagnation. If sincerely carried out, the act of noticing and consciously negating each and every hopeful thought to cross her mind may be enough to release the woman from Sepia's mind/body bind. Paradoxical, "prescribe-the-symptom" recommendations of this sort have been pioneered by logotherapists of the Viktor Frankl school[4] who routinely apply counterintuitive (but homeopathically analogous) stratagems in order to liberate their patients from self-imposed and self-reinforcing binds.

We might now look at how the work of the constitutional homeopath and the clinical therapist intersect. Both professionals are likely to view identification of a debilitating paradox that is central to a client's life and history as a core objective. A difference in methodology, however, between homeopaths and therapists becomes apparent: while homeopaths survey and investigate the full range of mental, emotional, and physical symptoms, therapists—despite ample possession of the interpretive knack—may limit their attention to a client's cognition, behavior, and affect.

Another difference: although a therapist investigates the background history in which her patient's complaint or disorder is rooted, the therapist may feel compelled to view, for example, anxiety or depression as separable from its context. For this reason, she may provoke a defensive reaction in her client. For the homeopath, however, it is immaterial whether an environmental circumstance promotes a particular remedy state or whether the same circumstance merely reflects the remedy state. The homeopath is also not constrained from accepting as legitimate any explanation a patient offers as responsible for initiating the disorder.

One of the purposes of this book is to provide therapists and caregivers an opportunity to extend the scope of their attention to, and understanding of, somatic symptoms. As will be repeatedly demonstrated, physical symptoms are a language aching to be decoded. Whenever somatic decoding takes place, the benefit to clinician and patient alike is self-evident.

Rather than supplying a case file, the following example of cure by means of prescribing the symptom is taken from a public event. It concerns the chronic illness of a renowned Boston baseball franchise stricken with a debilitating condition known as "The Curse of the Bambino." The Boston Red Sox could not win a World Series after basically giving away to the New York Yankees, for a piddling amount of cash, Babe Ruth, who, as it turned out, would become widely recognized as the greatest player in the history of baseball. In 2004, with the Red Sox team's miraculous, come-from-behind win in a playoff against the Yankees, and their subsequent rout of the National League's St. Louis Cardinals, the infamous curse was finally, after 86 years, put to rest. What had effected the cure?

The power of the curse was not mystical. Rather, it represented an entrenched fear and its related behavioral rigidity. States of "stuckness" just like this are routinely identified by classical homeopaths as "underlying illness states." The fear underlying "The Curse of the Bambino" was that team management might some day again commit an error as egregious as giving away Babe Ruth, the great Bambino. The rigidity was associated with the fear of making any baseball trades that were even remotely suggestive of this possibility. When installed as a core front-office belief, the fear delimited managerial flexibility, thereby placing the team at a disadvantage with respect to trading players with other teams.

There is in baseball a shibboleth that the value of even a handful of good players cannot equate that of a single great player. The reason for this is that truly great players are irreplaceable, while many even very good players can be readily exchanged for others of equal value. Avoidance of any such trade would be fully in keeping with the fear and rigidity associated with the Curse of the Bambino. In accordance with the homeopathic Law of Similars, however, the way out of an ideé fixe demands grappling with the original error (but only in a microdosage form). Yes, facing down the demon is better than doing nothing.

The Red Sox shortstop Nomar Garciaparra had been anointed the greatest Red Sox player since Ted Williams by no less a luminary than Ted Williams himself. Yet, in 2004, General Manager Theo Epstein was inspired to trade the irreplaceable Garciaparra for three talented but lesser lights. The day on which the trade was announced talk-show radio hosts went berserk. The trade was denounced in the newspapers as another Babe Ruth giveaway.

One can say, of course, that the team's chemistry improved because of the three new players, each of whom went on to play significant roles in the team's 2004 triumph. I would argue, however, that it was Epstein's fear-dispelling moxie that cured the curse and restored the franchise to health.

Recognizing Pathology By Level and Stage of Life Through Sense-dimensional Analysis

As shown in **Table 2**, in TCM each of the Five Phases and sense dimensions correlates with a specific stage of life as well as a level of pathology. Though this is an imperfect means of categorizing illness, the correspondences of life-stage and level of pathology with the five sense dimensions can be striking.

1) *The Dimension of Touch.* Touch is generally involved in transient symptoms such as fever and childhood terror which, though they may be severe, are superficially rooted. Accordingly, a quick-acting remedy such as Belladonna is often indicated. The following example concerns not only an adult pathology, but also a situation involving not transient but chronic symptoms. The condition nevertheless pertains to the dimension of touch.

Months after having undergone exhausting and arduous labor in delivering her baby, a young mother becomes afflicted with a terrifying and seemingly life-threatening panic disorder. The rapidly-acting remedy Aconite can express the element of terror within ailments associated with the core issue of synchrony versus isolation in the dimension of touch. If a single, high-potency dose of Aconite produces a cathartic resolution of the panic disorder, the indication is that her condition is not deeply rooted and may be located within the dimension of touch.

2) *The Dimension of Taste.* Taste includes a variety of ailments generally originating in adolescence, a time when anxiety is ordinarily more powerfully expressed than is challenge; anxiety and challenge are the opposing poles on the axis of the core issue in the taste dimension. Within taste, many anxiety disorders and metabolic conditions display acute symptoms such as fever, vomiting, chills, and muscle ache; but, although acute, they are more deeply rooted than symptoms associated with the dimension of touch. Examples of homeopathic remedies for anxiety within the taste dimension are Lycopodium clavatum and Graphites.

3) *The Dimension of Smell.* To the extent that we tend not to experience profound grief until adulthood, the dimension of smell relates to the adult life-stage. Conditions that are more deeply entrenched than those of the dimension of taste may occur again and again. When disorientation overcomes centeredness—the core issues within the smell dimension—periodically recurring depressions may be experienced on the anniversary of a loss or during the periodicity of seasonal affective disorder (SAD). A typical homeopathic smell-dimension remedy is Natrum muriaticum.

4) *The Dimension of Hearing.* The hearing dimension, expressive of the interplay between the two poles of entropy and consolidation, pertains to middle age, the life-stage when miasms, susceptibilities to illness, and genetic conditions often manifest; these conditions are much more deeply entrenched than are the symptoms associated with any of the previous dimensions. To the extent to which consolidated illness can undergo a catharsis and a cure, the homeopathic remedy Calcarea carbonica is a good fit with hearing. Also indicated are the Lanthanides of the periodic table of elements, and miasmatic remedies, many of which are nosodes.

Inherited congenital conditions such as amyotrophic lateral sclerosis (ALS) and cystic fibrosis are examples of core issues within the dimension of hearing that may be entirely refractory to emotional catharsis and to a cure. This does not mean, however, that congenitally afflicted individuals fail to derive benefit from any type of care. The practitioner will recognize that constantly working with the patient on the problematic aspects of an inherited condition represents a spiritually enriching process for the patient. Creating a partnership with the patient in this effort is a sufficient and even noble goal.

5) *The Dimension of Sight.* Insofar as ailments such as musculoskeletal stiffness and neurological conditions associated with stroke, palsy, and blindness manifest the dimension of sight's core issue of chaos overriding creativity, sight's correspondence to the stage of old age/death is evident. Cuprum and Zincum, indicated for seizure disorders, are examples of homeopathic remedies used within the dimension of sight.

Catalyzing Advancement in Spiritual Development

As will be shown in the following chapters, successful resolution of the core issues embedded within each of the five sense dimensions is associated with soundness of mental, emotional, and physical health. The degree to which such resolutions are complete or incomplete can be modelled schematically. Within Chapter 9, "Encountering Charybdis: The Chronic Illness Vortex," the energy dynamics and conditions of health and illness are found organized within and according to Five Phases-based, cyclical arrangements of the sense dimensions.

Having enlarged our focus, built our framework, and prepared for a journey beyond the bounds of biomedicine, the stage is now set for our entry into the domain of the five sense dimensions. Bear in mind that this book is a primer, a step-by-step introduction to the five sense dimensions. For this reason, illnesses have been selected for study that define and elucidate the sense dimensions while the study of the sense dimensions reveals new depths and wider horizons of chronic illnesses.

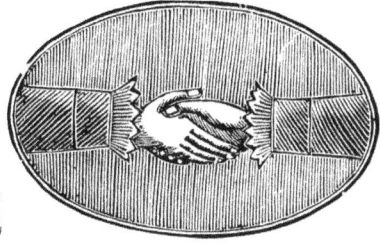

CHAPTER THREE

THE DIMENSION OF TOUCH

THE SENSE DIMENSION OF TOUCH

PHASE	FIRE
ORGAN	HEART
CORE ISSUE	SYNCHRONY-ISOLATION

Touch is the constellation of sensations that conveys pressure, heat, cold, torque, and pain. It is the most broadly distributed of the sense organs. But touch is not merely a passive receptor reporting conditions on the skin. Behind touch is the will to know and to be known, to commune and to communicate, to be in touch. This constitutes a call, with sensory inputs as the response. Call and response are exemplified by each contraction and relaxation of the heart, and by the cyclical departures and returns of circulating blood. Thus touch and the heart share a similar dynamic. When call and response are most meaningful, the heart has been touched.

A pattern of repeated calls and responses constitutes a cycle, a circular flow, circulation. It may be spoken of as a Great Return, as when the fresh rains eventually seep into a river and return to the salty sea. Vast herds and flocks migrate on epic journeys; a homing instinct draws them away and then back to their ancestral places. We may think similarly of the departure and long-awaited return of an exile. Not all circular patterns are positive: consider the deceptive self-limitation set up by some circular thought patterns, dangerous as a whirlpool's eddies. Thus the blockage of healthful cycles, the negation of essential return, underlies much that manifests as chronic illness.

Touch bridges separation by conveying the feel of others, letting us internalize the forms of the palpable world. That internalization structures the self in synchrony with the world. Martin Buber expressed synchrony as an "I-Thou" relationship, recognizing the profound kinship of the Self and Other. This same understanding is articulated in the ancient Vedic tradition with the phrase "Thou Art That." Touch is the medium of such profound linkages that we consider it to be the master of all other sense dimensions.

A study by Hertenstein and associates[1] at DePauw University, published in August 2009, indicated that even a touch between persons previously unknown to each other could accurately convey a specific emotion from one to the other. The study included a sample of 248 U.S. students, who were first blindfolded and then asked to silently touch or be touched on any appropriate part of the body by an unknown male or female partner and to convey by the touch one of eight specific emotions. The results showed that the rate of accuracy in reading the emotion conveyed by this touch ranged from 50% to 78%, much higher than the 11% expected by chance, and comparable to the rates shown in studies conveying verbal and facial emotions.

Touch bridges separation, yet touch can also establish separateness, informing us of otherness, of the not-self. This gap between the self and the other is the essence of isolation. Failure to call and failure to respond widen into a chasm of isolation. Isolation and the lack of touch foster anxiety. Ailments within the sense dimension of touch often have their origins in the shocking disconnection associated with heartbreak.

As skin is bridged by touch, one might expect skin diseases to be related to touch. In TCM, however, the Lungs are said to be the primary organ associated with skin diseases. Further, neurological disorders affecting the various touch receptors are more closely associated in TCM with the Kidneys when their locus is the central nervous system. Alternatively, they are associated with the Liver when their locus is the peripheral nervous system. More generally, a sense dimension in TCM is associated with an Organ and a Phase in relation to the experience of phenomena, and not through the physiologic transmission of stimuli.

At the end of this chapter are listed personal therapeutic practices designed to maintain the dimension of touch. Among these is drumming. If we had not understood that the call and response of successive drumbeats linked percussion with touch, we would have expected drumming to be classified with hearing. Our analysis of this hearing-touch synesthesia has been supported by a series of experiments reported by Gick and Derrick,[2] in 2009, in the journal *Nature*. The article indicated that the act of listening involves not only the ears but also the sense of touch. Moreover, sensations of touch were found to enhance what was perceived through the ears.

THE HEART IN TRADITIONAL CHINESE MEDICINE

In TCM the Heart is conceived of as the master of blood and its channels. It is also the residence of the spirit or mind, and so it is more accurate to refer to this organ as the Heart/Mind. The Heart and its paired organ, the Small Intestine, belong to the Phase (or Element) of Fire. Fire generates fever, heat, redness, and agitation when it is excessive. Pallor, coldness, or aversion to cold appear when it is deficient. Note that the Kidneys, though pertaining to the Phase of Water, also have an accessory Fire function. See Chapter 9 for a discussion of Phase relationships.

Although the Heart is the master of blood, in TCM two other organs provide important related functions. The Liver is the storehouse of blood and contributes to blood's smooth distribution. The Spleen is charged with keeping blood in its correct pathways. Problems such as hypertension or painful menses may involve the Heart, Liver, Spleen, and/or Kidneys.

Symptoms of Heart disharmonies in TCM include weak or irregular pulse, coldness, cyanosis, insomnia, anxiety, emotional instability, depression, agitation, and various manias. Biomedical diagnoses could include arrhythmia, angina pectoris, arteriosclerosis, anemia, hypertension, edema, epilepsy, stroke sequellae, neurosis, depression, bipolar disorder, and psychosis.

TOUCH DIMENSION CORE ISSUE:
THE SYNCHRONY-ISOLATION AXIS

SYNCHRONY

Synchrony manifests throughout the universe at every level and scale of existence. Electrons can act in concert as coupled oscillators, while in the macrocosm the planets make synchronous orbits around their stars and the moons around their planets. As noted by Huygens in the 17th century, two pendulums suspended from a single beam will, under certain conditions, adjust to swing consistently in opposite directions. A flock of birds on the wing will all at once shift direction without crashing together. Fireflies flash in unison by the thousands. Social trends and mass hysteria likewise flash into existence; medieval scientists would not have been surprised by such phenomena, as they expected a synchronous universe.

The emerging science of synchrony described by Steven Strogatz in his book, *SYNC: The Emerging Science of Spontaneous Order*,[3] suggests that the central mechanism operating within living things is a biological clock. This clock keeps time to a cyclical pattern, such as a circadian rhythm, that organizes the unfolding of biological activity. An organism can then be conceived of as a network of biological clocks that have evolved to behave in synchrony with one another. Thus, living things cluster purposively in time, whether they are cells forming tissue, bison running in a herd, fish swimming in a school, or human beings living in a community. Incidents of spontaneous healing are manifestations of supersynchrony, the outbreak of a powerful insistence on the integrity of an organic system.

Synchrony may be broadly defined as an activity rhythmically driven on behalf of a unification of purpose. Synchrony is the generator of common purpose, the organizational principle behind animate and inanimate creation. It is a fundamental expression of love that runs throughout creation. At the sensory level, it begins with the touch of skin with a separate entity.

Synchrony is typically healthful when it engenders bonding among individuals and communion with the greater wholes of community, ecosystem, and spiritual domain. We experience synchrony in group-identification, falling in love, being sucked into the flow of traffic in a rotary, and joining in applause even without appreciating a performance. But synchrony is not always a sign of health. Cancer cells cluster synchronously into a tumor. Crowds may turn riotous. At times when the individual voice is essential, it may not be heard, or worse yet, may not be offered. The self can become lost in the other, just as it also can become lost in isolation from the other. Extreme synchrony turns into its opposite, isolation.

Synchrony manifests at multiple levels. An inferior level of synchrony may compete with a superior level for our allegiance. Rejection of the synchronic pull of a righteous yet violent political movement may mean that one has chosen to act in synchrony with a higher level of love for humanity, God, or goodness. Typically, identification with an inappropriate level of synchrony is problematic, rather than being a simple deficiency or excess of synchrony.

ISOLATION

If synchrony is the positive pole of the synchrony-isolation axis, then isolation is the negative pole. Isolation is characterized by being out of touch, out of step, not in rhythm, and unable to act for a common purpose. Isolation would be the fate of a totally freestanding individual, if such an entity were ever to exist. Isolation is found at the root of many psychological ills considered in TCM as pathologies of the Heart. It is overcome, literally and metaphorically, through touch, through a rebinding of the individual in relationships that both honor and exceed the self.

THE HEART AND SYNCHRONY IN BIOMEDICINE

Our association of the heart with the call and response of synchrony bears closer examination from a biomedical perspective. If blood and oxygen are reduced, the heart responds to that call by down-regulating its own energy needs. The three coronary arteries, an extension of the heart, also cooperate with one another. If the progress of arterial blockage in one artery does not occur too quickly, the communicating branches compensate by gradually widening.

A slightly variable heartbeat is actually healthier than one steady as a metronome. An unvarying rhythm represents rigidity, tension, and an overly circumscribed response to stress. Coordination of emotions, cardiovascular reactions, and brain states has been demonstrated in mothers and their infants, in marital partners arguing, and among people in meetings. The poetical heart and the cardiological heart beat as one and the same. We continuously feel the heart as it beats.

At the level of the brain (the physical basis of the Mind portion of Heart/Mind in TCM) we find another startling example of synchrony in the function of mirror neurons. These neurons fire when an individual performs a task; they also fire when the individual observes another person performing the task. Mirror neurons let us track the intentions and emotional content invested in the actions of other individuals. This capability not only facilitates but foreordains social bonding, rapport, cooperation, and harmonious action.

TOUCH DIMENSION: CHRONIC ILLNESSES

TOUCH DIMENSION ILLNESS: EDEMA

Edema—swelling from the pooling of fluids—is caused by an increase in hydrostatic and/or osmotic pressure occurring in the microvasculature or interstitial areas. It may be the result of inflammation, congestive heart failure, or impaired kidney function. Edema from congestive heart failure clearly relates to the Heart, while edema from inflammation pertains to the sense dimension of touch. We will discuss edema's relationship to touch from the perspective of homeopathy, distinguishing among three remedies: Apis, Bovista, and Hamamelis.

TOUCH DIMENSION ILLNESS: EDEMA
HOMEOPATHIC REMEDIES

Apis: "Be Fruitful or Multiply"

Apis is made from honeybee venom; its effects mirror the natural history of the bee, bent on work or reproduction. Apis treats edema in cases in which there is a strong underlying conflict between work and reproduction, between being fruitful and multiplying. The patient seeks synchrony among, and benefit for, current family members; but this choice is frequently a conflicted one, and if unresolved, the conflict promotes pathology. Recent widowhood, the need to care for an ill parent, or a financial setback can serve as a shock that initiates an Apis state. In addition to edema, physical symptoms of Apis may include urticaria, cystic ovaries, hardening of the skin, restlessness, shortness of breath, stinging pains, and aggravation from heat.

As with a bee sting, the Apis picture's edema is the consequence of an inflammatory reaction. What is in Apis that connects the phenomenon of inflammation with problematic fertility? The answer appears to be an inflammatory enzyme, hyaluronidase, which is coincidentally present within both bee venom and the acrosome (or "warhead" of a sperm). Contact with hyaluronidase in fact, is what breaches the ovum's membrane and gains the sperm's entrance to the egg.

The radical disjunct here is that the desire to reproduce promotes the need to set limits on family size.

Bovista: "Big-Hearted Vulnerability"

Bovista (puffball) treats generalized, superficial edema, in which the pressure of the thumb against the skin will leave an indentation. The most telling characteristic of an individual who fits the Bovista remedy state is his openhearted and unreserved disclosures, even revealing the most intimate topics. When his forthright revelations are used against him, he reacts by being even more open and honest; his attempts to withhold information bring out awkwardness and stammering. He may feel puffed out, larger than he is, and awkward. He may misperceive objects in space and drop things. Other physical symptoms include vertigo, urticaria from excitement, a tendency to hemorrhage, palpitations, and a sense of having an enlarged heart.

By means of a puffy outer layer of edematous insulation, the subconscious seeks to shield the patient from harm. This damp protective layer disrupts surface circulation, producing skin that is also prone to warts, herpetic eruptions, and itching. The radical disjunct is that excessive intimacy promotes insularity.

Hamamelis: "I Get No Respect"

Hamamelis (witch hazel) treats edema of a venous nature: phlebitis, hemorrhoids, varicose distension, bruising, and soreness from injuries. Individuals who fit this remedy believe they fail to receive their due respect and tend to disregard the tribulations that are encountered in daily toil. That disregard allows difficulties to exact a greater toll than they would otherwise, leaving the individuals feeling cheated. These patients tend to place great stock in elevated and subtle conversation and to state their thoughts with great care. They can be bothered by disorder and yet they are indifferent to workaday business.

In venous congestion, the walls of blood vessels become knotted and hard. Within varicosities, fluids accumulate and blood stagnates: vessels bulge and swell, hindering the transport of deoxygenated blood back to the heart. What single consideration connects these mental, emotional, and physical presentations? Venous circulation, operating at a lower pressure is intrinsically less efficient than arterial circulation. Hence venous return is more of a burden and is subject to stagnation. The tendency is augmented when trauma is present.

Physical injury—specifically hemorrhage, which lowers blood pressure—increases the burden of venous circulation, promoting symptoms that share a common quality of sinking down. The radical disjunct at work here is that acting as if we are above tribulations unwittingly invites being dragged down by them.

TOUCH DIMENSION ILLNESSES: CARDIOVASCULAR DISEASES

A series of chronic cardiovascular diseases are associated with the dimension of touch: atherosclerosis, arrhythmia, and hypertension. Atherosclerosis relates directly to Heart as conceived in TCM, while arrhythmia and hypertension may also bear the strong imprint of other organs.

TOUCH DIMENSION ILLNESS: ATHEROSCLEROSIS

In the United States and the majority of Western countries, atherosclerosis is among the leading causes of illness and death. The condition afflicts the inner lining of the arteries, where cholesterol, cellular waste products, and fibrin are deposited, causing inflammation and eventually calcification. The arteries harden and narrow, leading to high blood pressure and increased risk of stroke and heart attack. Two homeopathic remedy states are distinguished for atherosclerosis: Cactus grandiflora and Baryta iodata.

TOUCH DIMENSION ILLNESS: ATHEROSCLEROSIS
HOMEOPATHIC REMEDIES

Cactus grandiflora: "My Heart is Crushed"

Cactus grandiflora (night-blooming cereus) is used when the keynote physical symptom is a feeling of tightness in the chest, like a hoop of iron constricting the heart. Disappointment in love, or trauma from overidentification with a suddenly separated person, can establish the emotional conditions of the syndrome. The heart continues to strive to go out to the loved one who is no longer there, producing a constricted or bursting sensation in the chest. We have on several occasions heard the refrain: "At night I pace around the house like a caged animal."

A related emotional presentation is produced by a breakdown in trust, such as can occur when one is treated unfairly in the workplace. The Whitehall II Study published in 2005 in the *Archives of Internal Medicine*,[4] reported a higher incidence of angina, heart attack, or death from coronary artery disease among workers who perceived a low level of workplace justice, compared with those who sensed a high level of workplace justice.

Some people deal with broken trust alone, constricting the natural warmth of the heart in isolation. This pattern reflects features of the cactus, whose thick and prickly skin discourages commerce with other living things. The plant blooms in the dark of night. In his work, *Some Cactaceae in Homeopathic Medicine*, Dr. Massimo Mangialavori identified a feature specific to cactaceae that even more profoundly expresses isolation within the touch dimension: he observed a state of absolute self-sufficiency to the point of doggedly resisting care among those he treated who were in need of cactus remedies.[5]

On the physical plane, both of the above presentations foster blood stagnation and heat. From a TCM perspective, contributing factors include excessive ingestion of fried and overly-heated foods. The radical disjunct is that subjugation of the heart's warmth invites uncontrolled heat within the heart's vessels.

The effectiveness of Cactus grandiflora as a heart tonic arises in some measure from its stealthy slowness of action. Gradual repair of the arterial wall helps to protect the stiff vessels from rupture. This cactus plant encounters intense desert heat and prevents excessive evaporation of its life-sustaining mucilaginous sap.

Baryta iodata: "Mocked Because Supply Lines Have Been Cut"

The Baryta iodata (iodide of barium) variant of atherosclerosis is characterized emotionally by a sense of helplessness in the face of loss of power. There is a paralyzing self-consciousness, accompanied by restless desperation and the delusion that one is utterly unsupported. The psychological stance is that of being mocked for being isolated and starved for support. In addition to physical symptoms of atherosclerosis, symptoms of thyroid disorder may also be present. In his book, *Homeopathy and the Elements,*[6] Jan Scholten recommends using Baryta iodata to treat atherosclerosis. The radical disjunct may be expressed as "the very fact that I appear on the world stage proves my powerlessness to exert a right to exist."

TOUCH DIMENSION ILLNESS: CARDIAC ARRHYTHMIA

Cardiac arrhythmia (or dysrhythmia) refers to irregularities in the heartbeat. The beat may be too fast, too slow, transiently irregular, or persistently irregular; the effects range from negligible to life-threatening. Stagnant heart blood and deficient heart blood can also cause palpitations.

In TCM an irregular heartbeat is accounted for as deficient Heart Qi or deficient Heart Yang. Digitalis and Lobelia inflata are the remedies indicated for the patterns of deficient Heart Qi and Heart Yang.

TOUCH DIMENSION ILLNESS: CARDIAC ARRHYTHMIA
HOMEOPATHIC REMEDIES

Digitalis: "What Does the Future Hold For Me?"

Digitalis is made from foxglove. In biomedicine, pharmacological doses of digitalis are used to strengthen and slow the heartbeat. In homeopathy, doses are given for an irregular heartbeat, especially in relation to mitral disease. In these cases, the pulse may be slow, intermittent, weak, and thready. Digitalis is also used when the least movement provokes violent palpitations and a feeling that the heart will cease to beat

Deficient Heart Qi indicates diminished functional energy of the heart. On the psychological plane, the patient experiences extreme fear, sadness over trifles, a readiness to be discouraged, despondency about the future, and suspiciousness; these feelings promote or reflect isolation winning out over synchrony within the dimension of touch. Physical symptoms include palpitations, shortness of breath on exertion, sweating, pale complexion, fatigue, weakness, and listlessness. The tongue will be pale and may have a deeply fissured center and swelling on either side. The pulse has a vacuous (in TCM, "empty") quality.

The radical disjunct may be expressed as the desire to know the future promotes or reflects a wish not to know what the future holds.

Lobelia inflata: "In Fear and Trembling"

Lobelia inflata (Indian tobacco) is a stimulating expectorant and respiratory relaxant and is considered toxic in high doses. In homeopathic doses, it addresses weakness of the pulse and the fear that the heart will cease to beat, along with symptoms of coldness. Deficient Heart Yang encompasses deficient Heart Qi, with the added feature of lack of vital warmth; additional physical symptoms include cold limbs or a generally cold sensation, and a bright and pale complexion. The tongue is pale, wet, and swollen; the pulse is deep, weak, or knotted. There may be a concurrent deficiency of Kidney Yang. The psychological profile includes hypochondria or "making a mountain out of a molehill." These characteristics promote or reflect isolation winning out against synchrony. The radical disjunct is that a desire for languor produces tension associated with fright.

Other homeopathic remedies of use in addressing cardiac arrhythmia include Crataegus and snake-venom remedies such as Lachesis, Crotalus cascavella, Crotalus horridus, and Naja tripudians.

TOUCH DIMENSION ILLNESS: HYPERTENSION

In biomedicine, hypertension is classified as primary or secondary. Primary hypertension—essential arterial hypertension—is of unknown cause and is responsible for over 90% of systemic hypertension cases. Secondary hypertension—elevated systemic blood pressure of known cause—comprises the remaining cases.

Although chronic hypertension affects the sense dimension of touch, it typically originates in other sense dimensions. TCM defines four syndromes that encompass the various symptoms of hypertension: hyperactive Liver Yang; turbid phlegm disturbing the head; deficient Kidney Essence; and a combined deficiency of Qi and blood. We will examine each in turn with their corresponding homeopathic remedies.

TOUCH DIMENSION ILLNESS: HYPERTENSION
HOMEOPATHIC REMEDIES

Bryonia: "I'm All Business"

Hypertension in the pattern of hyperactive Liver Yang is related to excessive worry or anger and the physical symptoms of headache or dizziness. Other symptoms include irritability, flushed face, tinnitus, dry mouth with a bitter taste, and dream-disturbed sleep. The tongue is red with a yellow coating, while the pulses are tight and rapid. The disharmony in this category of hypertension originates within the sense dimension of sight.

Closely fitting this pattern is the remedy Bryonia. Underlying the Liver Yang features listed above, Bryonia individuals are subject to bursting pains, an isolating overconcern with work, fear of poverty, homesickness, a tendency to be aggravated from movement (thus they are ameliorated by stillness), and when sleeping, a tendency to lie facing the wall. While not usually considered a foremost option in regard to hypertension, Bryonia's domain extends to the blood. The remedy state can include a bounding, forceful pulse, and alteration of the blood from congestion, with resulting persistent fevers. Thus, Bryonia must be considered to reflect or promote a hypertensive progenitor state.

Glonoinum: "I've Had It Up to Here!"

A patient presents a pattern of turbid phlegm disturbing the head, which includes symptoms of headache or dizziness, combined with a heavy and tight feeling in the head. The patient may also have a feeling of fullness and oppression over the chest and epigastrium, loss of appetite, and somnolence. The tongue is corpulent with a white greasy coating, while the pulses are soft and slippery. The pattern can result from improper diet, overwork, stress, or a protracted illness. Phlegm and dampness hinder the spleen and stomach functions of transporting and transforming nutrients. They also obstruct the ascent of pure Qi and the descent of turbid Yin. The disharmony in this category of hypertension originates within the sense dimension of taste.

The remedy Glonoinum, made from nitroglycerin, fits this pattern well. In keeping with the substance's pressurized and explosive character it is indicated in high blood pressure, especially in the elderly. Above and beyond symptoms following under the description of turbid phlegm, Glonoinum is indicated for a variety of head symptoms such as pulsation, a swollen and enlarged sensation, a feeling that the head could explode from pressure, sunstroke, and headaches from exposure to the sun. Specific features associated with dizziness include confusion and a lost sense of direction. Glonoinum's remedy picture promotes or reflects ailments arising from quarrelling and from aversion to one's spouse or children, features associated with the dimension of taste.

The Aurum Series: Remedies Coupling Deficient Heart and Kidney

The pattern of deficient Kidney Essence produces symptoms of headache or dizziness accompanied by an empty feeling in the head, tinnitus, weakness of the lower back and knees, impotence, nocturnal emissions, and a dry mouth. The tongue is red with a little coating, while the pulses are thready and weak. The disharmony in this category of hypertension originates within the sense dimension of touch, but its consolidated expression pertains to the dimension of hearing.

Jan Scholten, in his book, *Homeopathy and the Minerals*,[7] published in 1993, used a phenomenological technique, called group analysis, with which he predicted the profiles of as yet unknown homeopathic remedies. In a 1996 book, *Homeopathy and the Elements*,[6] Scholten enlarged his technique to predict the until now unproven homeopathic features of elements in the periodic table of elements according to what he called "element theory"—a "life-theme" analysis of the seven-fold horizontal arrangement of the elements as they intersect with the 18 stages associated with the table's vertical arrangement of the periodic system. The seven life themes, which correspond to the series of elements in each of the seven rows—for example, Row 1: hydrogen series (hydrogen and helium); Row 2: carbon series (lithium to neon); Row 3: silicon series (sodium to argon)—include, among others, individuality, family and relations, work, and creativity. In a subsequent book, *Secret Lanthanides*,[8] published in 2005, Scholten expanded his phenomenological exploration of the periodic table to a group of elements, the Lanthanides, that at one time were known as the rare earths.

Because of their ability to address imbalances conjointly involving the Heart and Kidneys, homeopathic remedies derived from the Aurum series of the periodic table—elements in Row 6, ranging from atomic numbers 55 (cesium) through 86 (radon), given the life theme "leadership and autonomy"—are especially important in treating hypertension that has features in common with TCM's description of deficient Kidney Essence (see **Table 1** on the following page).

Crataegus: "Pump It Up"

The pattern of deficiency of Qi and blood displays symptoms of headache or dizziness with lassitude, shortness of breath, palpitations, insomnia, and spontaneous

**Table 1. Characteristics of Homeopathic Remedies Derived
From the Aurum Series of the Periodic Table of Elements**

ELEMENT/ REMEDY	SOURCE	CHARACTERISTICS
Aurum	Gold	Tendency toward heart disease, depression, bone pain (associated with Kidney); sense of excessive responsibility; after traumatic heartbreak. Association with bipolar disorder.
Plumbum	Lead	Effects of high living; controlling nature, often very responsible position; suspicion of schemes. Association with neurological deficits.
Platina	Platinum	Mainly beneficial to women; after great loss or reversal of fortune; display of haughtiness, superiority, contempt for others. Association with numbness and hypersensitivity.

sweating. The tongue is pink with a thin white coating, while the pulses are tight and thready. Stress may impair the functions of the Heart and Spleen, causing Qi and blood to become deficient. The disharmony in this category of hypertension originates within the sense dimensions of touch and taste.

Crataegus, made from hawthorn, is a homeopathic heart tonic that appears to address symptoms closely approximated by Qi and blood deficiency. Additional and more specific features include apprehensiveness, despondency, nervousness, irritability, irregular and weak pulse, valvular murmur, pallor, and cold extremities.

Although we have suggested one homeopathic remedy, in complex cases exacerbated by cardiac disease, other remedies may be more appropriate. Likely to be of clinical use or worthy of study with regard to managing Qi and blood deficiency with hypertension are Lycopus virginicus, Digitalis, Kalmia latifolia, and Hydrocyanicum acidum.

TOUCH DIMENSION ILLNESSES: MENTAL DISORDERS

As previously noted, the Heart in TCM is truly the Heart/Mind. Mental disorders might therefore tend to be diagnosed in terms of the Heart. But every organ has a sense dimension, an emotional aspect, and emotional disturbances associated with it. From this stand-point, we offer an overview of alienation, bipolar disorder, hysteria, schizophrenia, and autism.

TCM theory posits a close relationship between the Heart and Mind and an aspect of consciousness known as the "Ethereal Soul," housed in the Liver. The Ethereal Soul is responsible for our life's creative energy and is most active at night in our dreams. When the mind stifles creativity, stagnancy and depression result. In mania, the Heart cannot sufficiently rein in the Ethereal Soul. Consequently, the Ethereal Soul invades the waking state and disrupts the mind's equilibrium. Depressive conditions thus reflect an imbalance of both Heart and Liver.

TOUCH DIMENSION ILLNESS: ALIENATION

Alienation (or disaffection) is a pervasive symptom, although it is not recognized as a freestanding syndrome in either TCM or biomedicine. Alienation is a type of isolation, and it fits squarely within the sense dimension of touch. We will describe three variants of alienation by their homeopathic remedies: Daphne mezereum, Kali bromatum, and Veratrum album. Each variant includes an aversion to touch and a range of symptoms involving the skin that reflects or predisposes a disaffected state of mind.

TOUCH DIMENSION ILLNESS: ALIENATION
HOMEOPATHIC REMEDIES

Daphne mezereum: "Dead to the World"

The chief psychological characteristic of Daphne mezereum is a feeling of dead emptiness, a disaffection in which no sensation is vivid. In addition, nauseous anxiety may be felt in one's stomach; one may feel quarrelsome, disorientated, a sense of stigmatization, and of being torn in one's loyalties; gestures may be false or affected. Physical symptoms have a violent and/or burning nature. A pathology of the skin is prominent, including itching and a feeling of ants crawling under the skin.

The pattern exemplifies suppression of a natural reaction to a toxic shock. For example, when the patient encounters an infuriating situation that admits of no response, he suppresses the natural expression of his anger. This suppression deadens the ego and contorts the inner world. The radical disjunct: accommodation of toxicity invites intolerance of toxicity. Daphne mezereum may therefore be used to offset the toxic effects of chemotherapy.

Kali bromatum: "God Hates Me"

Kali bromatum (potassium bromide) is used to treat disaffection that consists of paranoid delusions, a feeling of helplessness, insecurity, and a bad conscience. There may also be loss of memory and aphasia. Physical symptoms include numbness, impotence, fidgeting, a stumbling gait, prostration, and seizures. The skin may be afflicted with acne.

The sense of moral deficiency, of having been singled out by God for punishment, flourishes in the company of rigid puritanical values. Entry into this pattern of alienation may come from sudden anger, fright, emotional disturbance, business losses, embarrassment, sexual excess, or sexual abuse. The radical disjunct is expressed as excessive investment in moral uprightness promotes moral deficiency.

Veratrum album: "Only I Know the Way"

Veratrum album (white hellebore) is used for a disaffection that has a paradoxical appearance. The patient displays psychological characteristics of extreme haughtiness, relentless ambition, and self-righteousness. Yet he also suffers from severe and debilitating collapse, fear, a sudden sinking of strength, and immersion in meaningless and repetitive behaviors. Physical symptoms include sudden diarrhea, violent nausea, weakness, chilliness, and coldness of the stomach.

A person may enter this pattern after having had the rug pulled out from under him, or after a sudden trauma involving loss of position, place, or privileged state. The death or disappearance of a beloved parent may have a similar effect. This is the remedy for religious zealots and cult leaders. The radical disjunct can be stated as "I am so lost, only I know the right way!"

TOUCH DIMENSION ILLNESS: BIPOLAR DISORDER

Bipolar disorder, also known as manic-depression, encompasses dramatic mood swings ranging from unusual highs to extremely sad and despairing lows. Periods of normalcy can occur between these poles. We describe three variants with their homeopathic remedies: Aurum metalicum, Syphilinum, and Naja tripudians.

TOUCH DIMENSION ILLNESS: BIPOLAR DISORDER
HOMEOPATHIC REMEDIES

Aurum metalicum: "I Must Please God"

The psychological profile in this variant is that of an individual who takes on huge responsibilities. Although she is a high achiever, she never satisfies her personal standards of excellence. She is drawn to prayer or other forms of inner spiritual practice, seeking synchrony at the highest possible level. The depressive despair she can feel is usually attributable to a heartbreaking experience or loss. In the shattering of key associative bonds, the delusion of isolation is established. Physical manifestations include cardiac symptoms, high blood pressure, angina, palpitations, and pain described as issuing from deep within the bones. The radical disjunct pertains to a sense of self-worth that is linked to impossibly high standards of achievement: one must prove one's self-worth through achievements that are never sufficient. A manic redoubling of efforts to achieve more and more only produces exhaustion and greater despair, thereby establishing one's inherent worthlessness.

A constitutional predisposition to this type of bipolar disorder is attributed in homeopathy to the syphilitic miasm. Homeopathy's concept of miasm is equivalent to the concept in TCM that features of a congenital disease are imprinted onto the Kidney Yang. Symptoms of the syphilitic miasm include an unusual sense of struggle, intractable circular reasoning, and strong sexuality. The homeopathic remedy Syphilinum is often prescribed several weeks after Aurum metalicum, that is, after a depression has lifted significantly and the cardiac symptoms have been ameliorated. At this point, symptoms related to Syphilinum, previously in the background, become the focus of treatment.

Syphilinum: "Out Damned Spot!"

This variant of bipolar disorder presents as megalomania and rage against con-tamination, followed by a despairing sense of guilt. Mental symptoms treated by the Syphilinum nosode, made from a syphilitic discharge, include recursive logic, memory loss, and obsessive-compulsiveness often related to a germ phobia. Guilt, shame, isolation, and struggle are expressed in suicidal ideas and antisocial behaviors. Physical symptoms include prostration and putrefying abscesses and ulcerations. Sexual addiction may be a prominent feature.

In the miasmatic Syphilinum remedy state, an individual is caught up in a hopelessly circular desire for satisfaction. The core of that desire is sexual, whether the individual is aware of it or not. From the perspective of the sense dimension of touch, sexuality can be either isolating or synchronic. It is isolating when the physical act is not linked with an authentic emotional and spiritual meeting. The resulting emptiness then leads one to seek more sexual activity and possibly more partners. The radical disjunct is that physical sex devoid of emotional and spiritual fulfillment leads to ever more physical sex and greater emptiness. The desperation of sexual addiction perverts the interplay of closeness and apartness so character-istic of the world of touch.

Naja tripudians: "Capitulation to Guilt"

The core conflict in this variant, made from cobra venom, is a sense of being torn between two paths and deeply regretting a particular decision or pattern of be-havior. The individual suffers from an isolating sense of guilt for having neglected a duty. Long after the fact, he feels himself a failure and remains torn between two separate wills. At its most extreme, this duality can express itself in suicidal thoughts or behavior. Physical symptoms include palpitations and disorders of the heart valves. Other symptoms include choking respiration and hysterical mute-ness. The mania tends to be of a quiet sort, building on the delusion that the in-dividual must hold himself under superhuman control. The radical disjunct per-tains to excessive investment in one's situational responsibility, which then grows untenable. A split in the will develops, producing helpless capitulation to guilt.

TOUCH DIMENSION ILLNESS: HYSTERIA

In the analysis of mental disorders, the expression "hysteria" has been supplanted by the modern diagnostic term "conversion disorder," which refers to the conversion of psychological distress into physical symptoms. Because this kind of conversion applies broadly to so many medical conditions, we opt to use the older term, hysteria, within the context of this chapter.

Hysteria is erroneously linked only to females; in fact, both sexes are subject to this illness. Psychology texts connect the onset of hysteria with dissociation; this defense mechanism serves to protect the self after a traumatic event. The loss of connection that dissociation implies places it within the sense dimension of touch. Yet, as with all mental disorders, more than one sense dimension may be involved. For example, in the context of hysterical grief, Ignatia, which is the most highly regarded homeopathic remedy for hysteria, relates to the sense dimension of sight and will be covered later in that chapter of the book. Below are four variants of hysteria distinguished by their remedies: Belladonna, Hyoscyamus, Aconitum napellus, and Arnica montana.

TOUCH DIMENSION ILLNESS: HYSTERIA
HOMEOPATHIC REMEDIES

Belladonna: "Child's World"

The Belladonna (deadly nightshade) variant of hysteria includes nighttime terrors, oversensitivity, wild deliriums, furious rages, fits of laughter, teeth-grinding, fear of dogs, hallucinations, and a sense that one is dreaming while wide awake. Emotions flare with sudden and brief intensity. Various phobias are present--fear of having one's hair cut, or of the head becoming wet, or of exposure to the sun or wind, or of being shaken. The condition reflects the excessive imagination, sensitivities, and fears native to childhood. Physical symptoms include congestion and pulsation in the head and headaches. The radical disjunct here is that investment in freedom of the imagination promotes its opposite, isolation within a world too much one's own.

This variant provides TCM's perfect picture of the uprooted Ethereal Soul. Children are more prone than adults are to fall into this state; children are more imaginative, and the Ethereal Soul intrudes more easily into their consciousness.

Hyoscyamus niger: "Gaze on My Shame"

The Hyoscyamus niger (henbane) variant is characterized by shamelessness and exhibitionism. Symptoms include the inability to associate functionally, loquacity, suspiciousness, paranoia, and extreme silliness. On the physical plane the patient may have spasms, twitching, and a variety of nervous system disorders. There is a commingling of realms that normally do not touch, those of childhood bonds and of adult sexuality. Emotions issuing from breaking the unsophisticated rules governing childhood friendships are found to burst forth into the adult realm where they embody a lascivious parody of mature sexuality. The remedy's radical disjunct is that excessive investment in remaining as a child promotes the untenability of becoming an adult. A portrayal of this state may be found in the 1996 Australian film, *Shine*, based on the life of the pianist David Helfgott.[9]

Aconitum napellus: "Surely I Shall Die!"

The Aconitum napellus (monkshood) variant manifests as extreme anxiety and panic. Symptoms include terror and preoccupation with death, clairvoyance, extreme excitability, oversensitivity, and restlessness. Physical symptoms are intense thirst, tachycardia, oppressed respiration, numbness and tingling of the feet, weakness of the upper limbs, and sudden perspiration. Individuals in this pattern tend to have a desire for companionship, a marked fear of dissociation, and to be vivid and ruddy-faced. The radical disjunct is that overinvestment in the power to be strong and in circulation invites the opposite—terror and isolation.

The development of this condition signifies that one has had a sudden awareness of one's vulnerability, the acknowledgment of having absorbed a shock capable of knocking one out of circulation. This may result from a close encounter with death, such as surviving a crash or a harrowing childbirth.

Repeated low-potency dosing of the remedy can be sufficient to address a sudden onset of hysteria. Aconitum napellus is also useful for any illness that arrives with sudden acuteness. A very high potency is necessary to eliminate the panic and hysteria of a chronic or constitutional case.

Arnica montana: "The Hero"

In the Arnica montana (leopard's bane) variant of hysteria, there is not only the fear, but also the occurrence, of dissociation. The individual is dictatorial, quarrelsome, and obstinate. He is a know-it-all, taking strong issue with the opinions of others. He may feel himself to be an indestructible hero with important tasks to perform. Yet he is, if anything, a magnet for danger, subject to oversensitivity, a fear of being touched, and a delusion that he will die of heart disease. These individuals tend to be prone to hemorrhaging. The hysterical delirium is expressed in the certitude that all is well when, in fact, it is not. The radical disjunct is that overinvestment in one's muscular intactness invites excessive vulnerability.

Arnica montana is best known for treatment of acute muscular trauma and pain. Whether used in low potencies for this purpose or in high potencies to address hysteria, Arnica montana heals by making the inhabiting spirit feel at home.

TOUCH DIMENSION ILLNESS: SCHIZOPHRENIA

Schizophrenia was once known as dementia praecox, a name indicating organic brain deterioration in the young. In 1911, Swiss psychiatrist Eugen Bleuler coined the modern term, schizophrenia, locating the origin of the condition in disharmonious or contradictory tendencies in the mind, a split between thinking and feeling. It is now understood that schizophrenia contorts and consumes brain tissue while ravaging the personality and disorganizing the thought processes. Patients can experience disabling hallucinations, delusions, and deficits such as lack of speech, memory, expression, and affect. Although, in 1999, schizophrenia was reported to affect slightly more than 1% of the U.S. population,[10] the huge overall yearly cost of the disease in the U.S., in 2002, was estimated to be approximately $63 billion; the total indirect excess costs were estimated at over $32 billion.[11]

TOUCH DIMENSION ILLNESS: SCHIZOPHRENIA
HOMEOPATHIC REMEDY

Magnesia carbonica: "The Peacemaker"

The remedy Magnesia carbonica is indicated for severe mental instability. Its psychological profile is of a peacemaker who is highly sensitive to quarreling and who feels deeply unloved. This may stem from the shock of having witnessed heated or violent confrontations between parents at an early age. Terror of violence from others is paralleled by suppression of anger within one's self, which can destabilize the psyche. According to Edward Whitmont, "It [Magnesia carbonica] definitely would deserve a trial as a most promising drug in manic-depressive, as well as schizophrenic patients, whenever the symptoms agree."[12] The remedy's radical disjunct: the presence of others who are capable of nurturing and keeping one safe instead invites instability and danger.

SCHIZOPHRENIA AND CELIAC DISEASE

According to a population-based control study linked to Danish national registers conducted by researchers at Johns Hopkins University, in 2004, patients suffering from celiac disease were 3.2 times more likely to have been diagnosed with schizophrenia than were patients without celiac.[13] The sample population having both diseases, however, was very small, and other studies have not found a significant association between schizophrenia and celiac disease.[14,15] The Johns Hopkins study results suggested further study to see whether restricting gluten from the diets of the small proportion of schizophrenics who screen positive for celiac disease might help mitigate their mental symptoms. Modeling both diseases from the standpoint of TCM and homeopathy examines whether there is a possible association between the two diseases and suggests additional feasible treatments.

Celiac sprue is an autoimmune disease that involves a pathological reaction to gluten in which the hair-like, nutrient-absorbing villi of the small intestine flatten. Individuals suffering from celiac disease readily grow malnourished. They are also prone to other symptoms: indigestion, diarrhea, lactose intolerance, irritability, weight loss, bone pain, osteoporosis, anemia, dental problems, fatigue, thyroid disease, and neurological lesions similar to those found in multiple sclerosis. In 2002, a team of researchers led by investigators from Stanford University reported that a long-chain peptide that is a partially digested fragment of the gluten molecule is the likely trigger of the autoimmune response in celiac sprue.[16]

TCM has long recognized an association between the Shen (mental clarity) and the body's ability to absorb nutrients. The connection has to do with a "solid organ/hollow organ" relationship held to exist between the Heart and the Small Intestine. A diagnosis of "Full Heat in the Small Intestine" reflects a problem with the absorption of nutrients in the small intestine because of the retention of internal heat. This heat travels upwards in the body and disrupts the Shen. Symptoms that arise as a result of this action include mental restlessness, insomnia, tongue and mouth ulcers, pain in the throat, deafness, discomfort, heat in the chest, abdominal pain, and burning pain with urination.

TOUCH DIMENSION ILLNESSES: SCHIZOPHRENIA AND CELIAC DISEASE
HOMEOPATHIC REMEDY

Secale cornutum: "The Plight of Icarus"

Secale cornutum is made from a dilution of the parasitic Claviceps purpurea fungus found on grains such as rye and barley. Its ingestion via contaminated bread, for example, is responsible for a disease known as ergotism. Constituent ergot alkaloids not only constrict the smooth-muscle fibers and the walls of the small blood vessels, but are all to varying degrees psychoactive. One of these, a naturally occurring tetracyclic alkaloid, lysergic acid, is a source of the famous mind-expanding drug, lysergic acid diethylamide, or LSD.

Also known as St. Anthony's Fire, based on the agitated dance-like movements the condition produces, ergotism exhibits many features of acute schizophrenia. A possible outbreak of ergotism among the Puritans of New England at the time of the Salem witch trials is considered likely responsible for the epidemic paranoia and murderousness enacted upon women at that time. On the gainful side, a water extract of fermented barley was given by the ancient Greeks to Eleusian temple initiates in order to bring them into mystical states.

In parallel with TCM's diagnosis of "Full Heat in the Small Intestine," ergotism's hypersensitivity promotes mental restlessness as well as a disordered digestive function. Ergotism's physical symptoms manifest severe disharmony within the dimension of touch: unbearable skin sensitivity and hotness of the skin so severe as to culminate in numbness and even in gangrene of the extremities. Secale cornutum teaches a lesson similar to that taught to the mythical Icarus, who in his exuberance to fly came too close to the sun. If we seek to touch upon knowledge beyond our normal limits we risk searing our fingers. Ergotism's and Secale cornutum's radical disjunct may both be stated as "imprudent grasping after spiritual transcendence invites a spiritual crisis."

Of course, celiac disease manifests independently from schizophrenia. Because celiac's emergence among grain-dependent populations may be other than random, we hypothesize that hypersensitivity to cereal products proffers some evolutionary survival value: Because they are motivated to avoid grains, celiac individuals are more likely than the general population to survive even the most devastating outbreak of ergotism. The continued presence in society of celiac individuals may help protect the population at large from the delusionary and digestive ravages of ergotism.

TOUCH DIMENSION ILLNESS: AUTISM

To the extent to which susceptibility to autism or the autistic state itself is inherited, autism must be considered to have consolidated within the Kidney Yang and thus pertain to the dimension of hearing. Yet how does autism relate to the taxonomy of illnesses of the touch dimension? If alienation represents aversion to touch, then autism epitomizes being out of touch. This refers to the emotional impenetrability seen in autism, as well as the insensibility of a more physical nature. If intense physical stimulation is not provided, then autistic individuals are likely to feel nothing. Under the rubric of autism spectrum disorder, autism encompasses a variety of symptoms and a broad scope of social dysfunctions. We offer four symptom and variants of dysfunction by their homeopathic remedies: Mercurius, Helleborus, Tuberculinum, and Helium.

TOUCH DIMENSION ILLNESS: AUTISM
HOMEOPATHIC REMEDIES

Mercurius: "Terrifying Carnal Knowledge"

The Mercurius variant of autism manifests a mastery of communication linked with a destructive inability to access legitimate emotion. The patient may show a pervasive instability and a quicksilver changeability, perhaps accompanied by paranoia, anxiety, deceitfulness, timidity, extreme conservativeness, precocity, perversion, violence, and a desire to touch everything. The physical symptoms vary, potentially involving every tissue and organ in the body. One might see glandular inflammation, anemia, necrosis, congestion, edema, emaciation, tremors, or excessive sweating.

This syndrome mirrors the effects of sudden fear, as from a shocking sexual trauma. The radical disjunct may be said to be that an overly sudden introduction to intimacy (an excess of carnal knowledge) invites ignorance of true intimacy.

For several centuries, mercury compounds were a staple of Western medical care, widely administered in toxic pharmacological doses. Its use eventually became more focused on the treatment of syphilis and other sexually transmitted diseases (STDs). Homeopathic doses of mercury are similarly applied to STDs; Thuja occidentalis and/or Medorrhinum might also be used.

Mercury is a preserver that destroys all it contacts. Thimerosal, a preservative that has been used in vaccines, releases ethyl mercury as it is metabolized in the body. Given the large number of vaccinations that infants and children receive, there has been widespread concern over the potential for neurotoxicity and for neurodevelopmental harm from vaccine-related exposures to ethyl mercury. Manufacturers, urged on by the Food and Drug Administration, currently have developed thimerosal-free vaccines (or ones with trace amounts of less than one microgram/dose) for all routinely recommended childhood immunizations, other than inactivated influenza vaccine. For fetal protection, it is prudent for pregnant women to minimize exposures to mercury.

Helleborus: "See No Evil, Hear No Evil"

The Helleborus (Christmas Rose) variant of autism is best described as a sensorial depression, as if a veil covered each of the senses. This renders the individual slow to answer, gloomy, indifferent, and generally nonreactive. It takes every ounce of energy she may possess in order for her to perform a mental task. Physical symptoms include muscular weakness, sudden edematous swellings, and a slow, soft pulse.

This isolated state mirrors severe homesickness, disappointment, and heartbreaking neglect, as when a child is hospitalized but not visited by his parents—a symptom that can double as the radical disjunct: unhappiness in the presence of cheerful faces.

Tuberculinum: "Rebellion Within the Fortress"

The Tuberculinum variant of autism is characterized by rage and ritualistic behaviors. At its most extreme, the mental and emotional state also includes abusiveness, fits of temper, desire to travel, poor social contact, and romantic longings as unbearable as they are unquenchable. At its core, the individual's desire for freedom is juxtaposed with an imprisoning sense of enclosure. The radical disjunct: excessive demand for freedom invites imprisonment.

Tuberculinum is a nosode made from the tuberculosis mycobacterium. How can its actions on autistic rage and ritualistic behavior be explained? Autism's fortress-like impenetrability expresses the isolating effect of tubercular constriction and immobilization. Insofar as the alternating need to exert control and to break free underlies ritualistic behavior, Tuberculinum expresses relevance to vital force.

Helium: "Nothing Doing"

Helium is an inert gas located at the top right end of the periodic table of elements. In *Homeopathy and the Elements*,[6] Jan Scholten's discussion of this element provides a theoretical basis for the homeopathic use of Helium in autism. According to Scholten, Helium's elemental qualities consist of completion, retreat, and a cocoon-like state. The isolation and self-sufficiency of the autistic state are a close parallel.

Other key remedies used to treat autism that merit study include Bufo, Lycopodium, Cuprum metallicum, Agaricus muscarius, Kali bromatum, Stramonium, Carcinosin, Hyoscyamus, Opium, Syphilinum, and Tarentula hispania.

THE TOUCH DIMENSION: PERSONAL THERAPEUTIC PRACTICES AND MASTERS OF EXPRESSION

In addition to acupuncture, homeopathy, and biomedicine, various personal therapeutic practices promote health within the sense dimension of touch. **Table 2** lists a few of such practices.

A number of masters throughout history have powerfully expressed the positive and negative poles of the sense dimension of touch. **Table 3** lists several of these masters who exemplified one or the other side of the synchrony-isolation axis, the core issue of the touch dimension.

Table 2. Touch Dimension: Health-promoting Practices

Devotional practices	Reverence for origins
Massage	Poetry
Philanthropy	Drumming, dance, song
Yoga, Reiki	Spiritual involvement
Nurture the mother of touch, *Sight*: "Convert anger into creativity"	Environmental, social links

Table 3. Examples of Masters of the Sense Dimension of Touch

NEGATIVE POLE: ISOLATION	POSITIVE POLE: SYNCHRONY
Albert Camus	Martin Buber (I-Thou)
Sylvia Plath (*The Bell Jar*)	Steven Strogatz (*SYNC: The Emerging Science of Spontaneous Order*)
Charles Bukowski (disaffection)	Spiritual leaders, energy healers, Romantic poets

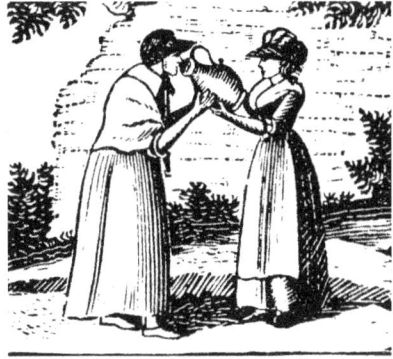

CHAPTER FOUR

THE DIMENSION OF TASTE

THE SENSE DIMENSION OF TASTE

PHASE	EARTH
ORGAN	SPLEEN AND STOMACH
CORE ISSUE	CHALLENGE–ANXIETY

Taste is the sensorial foundation of our ability to make distinctions. The Biblical tale indicates that when Adam and Eve tasted the apple, they were enabled to make distinctions between good and evil. The root word of sapience (wisdom, knowledge) is sapor (taste). Thus the sense dimension of taste is related to contemplation and thought.

Research evidence no longer supports the idea that the tongue contains a simple map of flavor receptors. All parts of the tongue's surface, in fact, can detect every flavor: 50 to 100 receptors appear to exist for each of the basic tastes and for considerable variation in individual taste. The tongue's chemical receptors delineate not only sweet, salty, sour, bitter, but also umami. Taking its name from Japanese, umami is a savory and is associated with meats, some cheeses, and mushrooms. Umami receptors are stimulated by monosodium glutamate, a taste-enhancing food additive.[1] In addition to these five tastes, the tongue may have chemical receptors for fat.[2]

Flavor is the combined assessment of taste, smell, and touch (texture and temperature). Memory also adds to the perception of flavor. Smell contributes greatly to the specificity of the identification of flavor; we can identify over 1,000 smells, but only a handful of tastes. That is why disturbances in the perception of flavor are mostly attributable to disorders related to smell. Dysfunction in the taste component of the perception of flavor may be caused by dryness of the mouth, oral infections, certain medications, radiation injury, burns, nutritional deficiencies, Bell's palsy, and dentures. Aging is a significant additional risk factor as it can reduce the acuity of both taste and smell.

THE SPLEEN IN TRADITIONAL CHINESE MEDICINE

In TCM the Spleen rules over the transformation of food and drink, separating the pure from the impure and then transporting these fractions through the body. This replenishes Qi and blood and nourishes the muscles. For this reason, the Spleen is said to rule the muscles and limbs. When the Spleen does not replenish Qi and blood sufficiently, fatigue and muscular atrophy occur.

The Spleen governs the blood, preventing hemorrhages by holding blood in its proper channels. The Spleen Yang is also thought to hold organs in position, preventing prolapses. The Spleen's transforming and transporting functions pertain to the production and movement of fluids in the body. These fluid functions contribute to and overlap with those of the Kidney. From a biomedical perspective, the Spleen in TCM incorporates the functions of the pancreas and also sweeps in the supply of cellular energy. The pancreas produces insulin to regulate blood sugar as well as digestive enzymes. The supply of cellular energy refers to cellular respiration, which produces carriers of chemical energy within cells.

The Spleen and its paired organ, the Stomach, belong to the Phase of Earth. The Phase of Earth is the postnatal foundation of health, as its organs supply the nutritive fractions that generate the Qi and blood necessary to sustain life and nourish all the other organs. For this reason, the Earth always occupies a central position in health and illness.

Besides hemorrhages and prolapses, symptoms of Spleen disharmonies in

TCM include edema, excess phlegm, cloudy urine, muscular atrophy, dizziness, seizures, fatigue, metabolic disorders, and a large number of digestive disorders. The loss of the sense of taste is a sign of disturbances of the Spleen.

TASTE DIMENSION CORE ISSUE: THE CHALLENGE–ANXIETY AXIS

Substances taken into the mouth as food have the potential to be either nutritive or toxic. There is a subtle and proper edge of anxiety in this venturing forth of taste, as the body meets and consumes or rejects foods. Taste is the first arbiter of the life-or-death digestive distinctions that we encounter with every bite.

Anxiety associated with taste in the act of eating is mirrored at another level by anxiety in the act of obtaining food. Whether in the hazards of the hunt or scrabbling through lean seasons, our dance with acquiring sustenance is inextricably linked with primal anxiety. The anxiety of obtaining food is experienced by every infant, newly dependent on external sources of food.

The functions ascribed to the Spleen in TCM include not only those that are digestive, but also those that supply cellular energy. The symptom of pervasive fatigue associated with the Spleen can be modeled at the level of the production of cellular energy. Producing cellular energy presents such significant challenges to the body that it has invested in backup systems to provide coverage in the event of failure or overload.

Mitochondria are the cell organelles that generate energy for cells. They produce chemical energy carriers, high-energy molecules such as adenosine triphosphate (ATP). Defects in ATP production may stem from abnormalities in nutrient uptake, in the Krebs cycle of aerobic reactions, in oxidative phosphorylation, or in errors of genetic signaling. Cumulative mitochondrial damage (as happens from chronic exposure to free radicals) contributes to fatigue, functional aging, and symptoms consistent with deficiency of the Spleen Qi.

When there are extreme energy demands, or when mitochondria fail, cells fall back on anaerobic metabolic pathways to generate high-energy molecules. Anaerobic metabolism is far less efficient than aerobic metabolism, but it allows us to survive, although just getting by. The organs most adversely impacted by mitochondrial disorders are the higher energy users. These include the brain, skeletal and cardiac muscle, sensory organs, and the kidney. Mitochondrial disorders are possibly at the root of chronic fatigue syndrome. The anaerobic backup system is an imperfect safety net, maintained against the uncertainties and high challenges of aerobic metabolism. It provides an example of the challenge-anxiety axis operating at the level of cellular biochemistry.

CHALLENGE

Anxiety, when it is accepted and invited, becomes challenge. Challenge is the psychological, biological, and material will to obtain mastery over anxiety. The hunt can be fearsome, or it can be taken as a tableau for exemplifying courageous adulthood. The grounds for challenge are also found in the process of eating. We sometimes bite off more than we can chew and then we must chew it over.

Once the body accepts a challenge, its biological response is to cash in one or more units of fuel currency, namely, the molecule ATP. A recent discovery with regard to the ATP molecule offers credibility to the concept that challenge is directly and immediately associated with the mouth. In addition to providing the body with fuel, ATP has now been found to perform yet another essential function, that of a nonneuronal "neurotransmitter" which conveys information regarding the sense perception of taste, as well as that of other senses. When released by nonneuronal cells like those found in the oral cavity, ATP triggers protective responses within the body that may build osseous tissue (bone) calculated to meet a challenge.[3]

The gut faces the considerable challenges of transporting ingested materials, breaking them down into absorbable forms, extracting nutrients, and ridding the body of waste products. At every stage in the carefully gated process of transport, breakdown, assimilation, and rejection, the potential for costly error is present. In health, anxieties do not overwhelm the challenges to achieve satiation, our repletion with the necessities of life itself.

ANXIETY

The anxiety that begins with taste makes itself known in the depths of the gut. The enteric nervous system is a brain within the lining of the gastrointestinal tract, extending from midesophagus to the anus. It has autonomous functions, but it is also connected with the central nervous system by the vagus nerve. Relying on the same neurotransmitters as the cranial brain, the enteric nervous system controls local blood flow, directs propulsion along the digestive tract, and may affect absorption. Under stress, it can shut down the digestive system or signal it to empty by means of excretion or vomiting. It can also trigger an immune response, causing mast cells to release histamine in the lining of the small intestine and colon. The enteric nervous system tastes the contents of the intestinal tract with chemoreceptors that react to acids, sugars, and amino acids. Our brain in the gut is thus charged with making key distinctions; it clearly recognizes the anxiety of fight-or-flight situations.[4]

The body's ability to perform expulsion is a functional aspect of anxiety. A judgment is made within the dimension of taste that a pathogen, a nonviable fetus, a transplanted organ, a morsel of food lodged in the esophagus, or an ingested toxin can no longer be accommodated or assimilated. The body then mobilizes to repel, or to expel, the substance with sneezes, coughs, gag reflexes, vomiting, and loss of motility in the bowel or uterus.

TASTE DIMENSION: CHRONIC ILLNESSES

More ailments pertain to the sense dimension of taste than to all other dimensions combined. We will provide examples of several of these ailments—generalized anxiety disorder, anorexia nervosa, arthritis, diabetes, chronic fatigue syndrome, and gastroesophageal reflux disease (GERD)—and describe homeopathic remedies for each, based on their ability to highlight the dimension of taste and their significant clinical usefulness.

TASTE DIMENSION ILLNESS: GENERALIZED ANXIETY DISORDER

Although no single homeopathic remedy perfectly fits the generic description of generalized anxiety disorder, numerous remedies exist that both describe and effectively treat specific nuances of anxiety. Generalized anxiety disorder may in fact be characterized by a range of symptoms:

- Exaggerated worry and tension, although provoked by little or nothing
- Constant anticipation of disaster
- Frequent excessive worry about health, money, family, or work

- Anxious thoughts of just getting through the day
- Physical symptoms, especially fatigue, headaches, muscle tension, muscle aches, difficulty swallowing, trembling, twitching, irritability, sweating, and hot flashes
- Light-headedness or shortness of breath
- Nauseated feelings or frequent need to go to the bathroom
- Inability to relax
- Startling more easily than other people
- Tendency to have difficulty concentrating
- Trouble falling or staying asleep

TASTE DIMENSION ILLNESS:
GENERALIZED ANXIETY DISORDER
HOMEOPATHIC REMEDIES

Lycopodium clavatum

Derived from club moss, Lycopodium is a famous polychrest, so-called because it correlates with a personality archetype and is one of the most tried and tested and most often used remedies in homeopathy. Lycopodium can be relied on to help profoundly insecure, distracted, and immature individuals.

Lycopodium patients manifest anxiety as a terror of public speaking. They can also experience anxiety in open spaces (which pushes their "I am insignificant" hot button) and in confined environments such as elevators that heighten a sense of being squeezed into a corner. Lycopodium individuals readily feel powerless. They manifest a sense of inadequacy that is compensated for by disproportionately controlling levels of behavior. Such individuals are given to practice martial arts, to bingeing on carbohydrates or sugar, but also to compensatory feats of radical dieting. The Lycopodium man or woman may be a coward or a bully or some combination of both. He or she is always a people pleaser.

In terms of the radical disjunct, the Lycopodium patient craves a challenge, although when provided with one, he feels overmatched or intimidated. His chief hot button is political, a delusion that even the most innocuous request is a command. In response he either buckles under or fights back like a cornered rat. The remedy state can disorder the gastrointestinal system, producing excessive gas and heartburn. It can also account for asthma and shortness of breath and compromise circulation, causing Reynaud's syndrome. It plays a role in a variety of reproductive complaints and, not surprisingly, in impotence and/or philandering.

Our familiarity with the typical gateway to the Lycopodium state sheds further light on the dimension of taste. Lycopodium teaches us the equivalence of empowerment, the acquisition of a core competence, and emotional security. A child about to be weaned from the breast, for example, must gain a core competence that is both frightening and empowering. In gaining awareness that his hunger is a separate and not always met need, he must grow adept in making the presence of hunger known. In addition the child must master ingestion of solid food. If the transition is at all traumatic, a feeling lingers that "I am not quite there yet. . . ." The infant's appetite then greatly enlarges; he becomes cranky and prone to colic.

A similar challenge awaits the child about to be toilet-trained or who is learning to read. The child's awareness of limited competence fuels an excess of self-awareness that further subverts his ability to enter into the flow of a competence-based activity. Subconsciously comparing his reading skills with those of another child, he is now distracted from the book in his hands. Failing to absorb its contents, he spirals more deeply into self-consciousness.

One of my patients, an extremely insecure and angry fourteen-year old girl offhandedly remarked that she first began having menstrual periods at the age of ten. In fact, early onset of menses is a Lycopodium keynote. For this girl, who at the age of ten was in no sense reproductively mature, menstrual precocity both signaled and predisposed her to a lasting Lycopodium remedy state.

A successful transition to a new core competence is immensely empowering. An incomplete transition, on the other hand, compounds self-consciousness, producing a lingering immaturity that reinforces one's delusion of incapability, and incomplete development becomes a self-fulfilling prophecy. It is fortunate that Lycopodium has proven to be such a handy weapon, not only against anxiety, but also against attention deficit disorder, reading disability, and a variety of appetite disorders.

Kali carbonicum

Derived from potassium carbonate, Kali carbonicum illustrates an aspect of TCM's understanding of the Spleen, an iconic organ related to Earth. The Spleen is responsible for the transportation and transformation of fluids. TCM theory also finds the Spleen to be either at fault for, or victimized by, obsessive thinking—an expression of anxiety. Moreover, dysfunction within the sense dimension of taste also can lead to obsessive thinking and repetitive thoughts.

According to the renowned homeopath Dr. Rajan Sankaran, a fear that one lacks the support of one's family represents the core theme of potassium-based remedies.[5] An unconscious fear that one is lacking familial support inflates challenge, thus provoking the anxiety found in this remedy.

You will often hear a Kali carb individual lament, "I can't believe she said that!" or, "I can't believe that so and so did such a thing!" He or she is ethically rigid and judgmental. In radical disjunct terms, the patient's desire for moral distinctions causes aggravation.

In addition to espousing black or white opinions, a person needing this remedy is predisposed to conservative views and is stressed by transitional or ethically unclear situations. The strong-minded barbs of an irritable Kali carb person are hurled inwardly as well as outwardly toward others. The individual is self-antagonistic, notably hard on himself. In accordance with enteric nervous system dictates, most of the related anxiety he or she experiences is felt in the stomach.

When a person is anxious, the mouth often becomes dry. Kali carb figures into this feature of fluid metabolism: the mental sphere is found to reflect dynamics within the physiological sphere and vice versa. We have already noted this remedy state's anxious, black-and-white mind-set. Its physiological equivalent is found in how moisture is processed within the mucous membranes. In normal functioning, the mucous membranes, whether they are found in the sinuses, the gut, or the endometrium, absorb accumulating moisture in a timely manner. In the Kali carb patient, however, the processing of moisture is other than timely. Moisture accumulating within the mucous membranes builds up until it can only be cleared by a violent allergic reaction such as a congestive cough or a sneeze. The mucous membranes thus tend to be either overly dry or congealed with viscid gunk. In TCM, this Kali carb state manifests as a Damp Phlegm disorder.

If Kali carb is indicated, so-called allergens must be held blameless for this condition. Instead, it is the length of time, induced by moral inflexibility, during which dander and pollen are mired in the mucous membranes that accounts for the allergic miseries, not the substances themselves.

Homeopathic materia medica suggests an indication for Kali carb among women having a history of first trimester miscarriage. Other clinical features, such as integrin growth factor, an adhesion molecule responsible for aiding fetal implantation within endothelial tissue, may also lead the practitioner to suspect a need for Kali carbonicum.

Kali carbonicum and arthritis

Although it is not included in the discussion of arthritis, Kali carbonicum possesses a particular affinity for the hip joint, which a patient's black-and-white mind-set inflames and renders arthritic over time. The Kali carb individual's exaggerated need to stand her ground in the face of real or strongly perceived opposition makes this association understandable. Under optimal conditions, the hip, comprising the body's largest joint, must figuratively and literally support one's stance in the world. Called on to provide both vertical and horizontal stability, the hip must provide a balance of firmness and flexibility. Standing overly firm, but hard-put to roll with the punches, the Kali carb individual is predisposed to back pain, sciatica, and arthritis of the hip.

Phosphorus

The second element in the periodic table's group 15, phosphorus has a glow that obscures its source, making it difficult to see where the substance begins and ends. Consistent with this feature, Phosphorus individuals have trouble setting boundaries, expressed in their tendency to hemorrhage (the blood does not remain within the capillaries), to connect too readily with strangers, and to manifest spaciness and scattered thinking. Key rubrics in which Phosphorus is prominent relate to oversensitivity to impressions, an artistic temperament, reactivity to thunderstorms, vibrancy, an appealing nature, and having a flair for color. Phosphorus individuals are susceptible to respiratory problems, hypoglycemia, prostration, and inflammation.

Phosphorus patients exhibit extreme anxiety, a counterbalancing reaction to having taken in too much. An understanding of the biochemical role of phosphorus illuminates this feature: along with hydrogen, oxygen, nitrogen, and carbon, phosphorus is one of only five elements constituting DNA, the genetic material of all living organisms. It is a key component of adenosine diphosphate (ADP), an ester of adenosine that is converted to adenosine triphosphate (ATP) for the storage of energy, and is the basic energy unit of aerobic metabolism. Phosphorylation, the introduction of a phosphate group into a molecule (the first stage in a reaction that can produce ATP) enables inert organic compounds to become biochemically active. Phosphorus is also required in the formation of bones and teeth.

What do these functions have in common and how might they relate to Phosphorus's radical disjunct? Phosphorus, which can be combustible, is intimately connected with the spark of life, to subtle events allowing inert matter to quicken. Without phosphorus, organic life cannot code or respire; muscles do not twitch. With phosphorus, heavily mineralized substances become tissue; teeth and bones acquire a living core.

Phosphorus's challenge is to maintain proximity to the source of creation; its anxiety is to avoid becoming apprehensive or frightened during this encounter.

Arsenicum album

Arsenic immediately follows phosphorus in the periodic table's group 15. In homeopathic microdosage, this deadly chemical is deservedly famous for its ability to reverse intractable anxiety. Underlying all anxiety encountered in Arsenicum patients is a preoccupation with, and fear of, death. Arsenicum individuals are fastidious, frugal, dependent on and enmeshed with their family and caregivers. They can be obsessed with health, disease, or aging and decay. Tending to be perfectionists and tormented by the possibility of error, Arsenicum individuals make excellent project coordinators and office managers who feel that "I am the one who reliably gets it done."

TASTE DIMENSION ILLNESS: ANOREXIA NERVOSA

The following case history illustrates some of the complexities inherent in an anorexia nervosa condition:

A patient of mine brought her thirteen-year-old, anorexic niece to me. The girl whom we will call Marta arrived with her parents who were uncommunicative in the course of the interview. Our session revealed a Marta who was polite, generous, and an outstanding student, with numerous devoted friends. Yet her dance teacher found herself compelled to remove her from performance rehearsals because Marta was displaying an alarming weight-loss to which she was indifferent. Apart from a delusional belief that she was overweight, Marta had few complaints, nor would she admit to any anxiety concerning death. Because Marta acknowledged having occasional stomach aches, I was able to question her about them. In a statement that I interpreted to reveal a fear-based and subconscious desire to return to the safety of the womb, she admitted, "My stomach can feel as if it is collapsing inward." I prescribed a high-potency dose of Arsenicum album.

In the weeks following, Marta's parents neither called me nor accepted my phone calls. I subsequently learned from her aunt that Marta had begun to eat normally and was gaining weight. At the same time, she had begun to vent uncharacteristic anger. The uncorking of Marta's anger apparently upset the ecology of her family; it appeared that so long as Marta did not speak up, dysfunctional family topics remained suppressed. The Arsenicum album I gave her, however, appeared to free Marta from her central role in support of this dreadful dynamic. It also revoked her delusional need to starve. Had Marta's parents kept an appointment for a second consultation, an accurate follow-up remedy would have helped Marta to process the root cause of her rage. Were it possible, I also would have referred the entire family for counseling.

TASTE DIMENSION ILLNESS: ANOREXIA NERVOSA
HOMEOPATHIC REMEDIES

Vanadium

Often indicated in cases involving anorexia and bulimia, the remedy Vanadium displays anxiety versus challenge to a prominent extent. Scholten[6] places the metallic element Vanadium in the ferrum series of the periodic table, where Vanadium's relationship to challenge reflects the ferrum series' general orientation toward work, duty, and control. Vanadium occupies the fifth position on the 18-stage cycle, the totality of whose arc Scholten identifies as extending from one's engagement with a project at its incipience, through a rise to the zenith of success regarding the project, followed by a gradual fall from prominence in relation to the work or project. The fifth state, identified with the last steps before one confidently assumes a project's ownership, features tantalizing susceptibilities toward postponement, self-doubt, overpreparation, and perfectionism. Stuck in the self-tormented, fifth-stage position, the Vanadium individual cannot help vacillating between ability and incapability with regard to the project.[6] How this conflict might translate into anorexia and bulimia is not difficult to comprehend.

Arsenicum album

Not surprisingly, Arsenicum album is efficacious in a variety of digestive complaints. It is almost a specific remedy for high-achieving, perfectionist school girls suffering from anorexia nervosa. The fathers of such girls are often demanding, exacting high standards of excellence, a circumstance that illuminates the nature of challenge within the remedy and its radical disjunct: "I crave a state of perfection so as to stave off death; but when I achieve this state, I perceive the stagnated nature of the perfected state, and this creates further terror of death."

TASTE DIMENSION ILLNESS: ARTHRITIS

To the extent to which susceptibility to this painful condition is not genetic, arthritis can be considered a metabolic ailment. What we choose to eat and how successfully our metabolism deals with the resulting challenge largely determines whether our joints become dull and achy, hot and inflamed, or swollen or stiff. The fact that anemia, an insufficiency of red blood cells, generally accompanies connective tissue disease lends credence to a link between arthritis and the malabsorption of nutrients that enrich the blood.

For our digestive system to remain well-toned, we need to maintain a steady diet of the fiber of raw fruits and vegetables. When deprived of this diet, the lower intestine becomes lax and prone to diverticula (outpocketings) and leakage, which subsequently produces a malabsorption cascade. As the intestinal walls grow increasingly prone to irritation and inflammation, they grow less able to tolerate normally fibrous fecal matter, and the need for a low-fiber diet escalates.

The digestive system needs the challenge of breaking down a wide variety of complex proteins and carbohydrates. A diet of overly processed foods creates gut-brain frustration in response to which underutilized enzymes, finding themselves deployed to the joints and synovial cavities in order to battle phantom pathogens, develop an autoimmune pattern of rheumatic inflammation and pain.

Unfortunately, it is not easy for us to maintain optimal diets. TCM as well as homeopathic materia medica are in agreement that fluctuation in emotional states such as one encounters during anxiety contributes to or reflects dietary choice. This has ramifications for arthritis. Within TCM there is no meaningful difference between a climatic pathogen such as Damp and its internal dampness counterpart. TCM theory describes internal pathogens which the Chinese term

"Evils" and which possess climatic features. The resolution of anxiety thus enhances one's ability to sustain a healthier pattern of eating that helps to promote a reversal of susceptibility to arthritis.

HOMEOPATHY, TCM, AND ARTHRITIS
HOMEOPATHIC REMEDIES

TCM describes arthritis pain in terms of a blockage or an obstruction occurring within energetic channels carrying Qi or Blood. Homeopathy sheds further light on the mental and emotional features that accompany an internally and externally caused pathology. Each of the following remedies illustrates a possible homeopathic response to a particular, well-known blockage.

Calcarea carbonica (Damp)

Having personally experienced and been made ill by the extraordinary humidity in the part of China I was staying in (I had an unusually nasty case of bronchitis), I can attest that Damp is more than a metaphoric descriptor. Also known as a Stationary Obstruction in TCM, Damp pertains to a fixed and localized pain, where the body and limbs feel heavy, often numb, with a tendency to edema. The constitutional picture of Calcarea carbonica (calcium carbonate) includes these characteristics and more. Calcarea individuals manifest a subtle defect that reflects the metabolic and generally binding significance of calcium, a result of which is that he or she easily gains weight and displays a tendency to clamminess or to suppression of sweat.

Calcarea carbonica is made from tortoise shell, an indicator of the Calcarea individual's placing a high premium on having adequate shelter and security. At its worst, the Calcarea individual's anxiety stems from a feeling that he is flying apart at the seams or going crazy, or that he lacks a single, overriding principle with which to explain his existence. He is given to entertaining metaphysical questions about life's purpose. A somatic and preverbal expression of this question, "When will it all come together for me?" is expressed in infants whose skull fontanels are tardy in knitting together.

Calcarea's radical disjunct becomes evident with respect to the remedy's challenge, that is, how the Calcarea individual tackles a project. He is inclined to process, analyze, and systematically break down a task into its constituent parts. On finding that there is a multitude of component parts, he becomes overwhelmed.

Being overwhelmed he applies himself even more systematically and analytically to the task at hand, thus spiraling his anxiety. After receiving a constitutional dose of Calcarea carbonica, an individual will likely find that his metabolism has become more effective. He will be able to lose weight, will generally feel warmer, and will be less prone to becoming overwhelmed, Moreover, the tendency to dampness (external) and swelling (internal dampness) decreases, significantly ameliorating arthritic pain.

Bryonia (Cold)

Also known in TCM as Painful Obstruction, Cold conditions are especially painful, made worse from exposure to climatic cold, and improved by exposure to warmth. When originating from outside the body, Cold has a contracting influence, inhibiting the flow of Qi and Blood, and tending to congeal fluids. Bryonia, which is made from wild hops, closely approximates this clinical picture with additional, illuminating specifics.

Bryonia individuals tend to be irritable, materialistic, and focused on their work. They are likely to fear poverty, which, according to homeopathic theory, reflects what is called the psoric miasm. Bryonia's anxiety and attitude toward challenge relates to a deep-seated ambivalence concerning dependence on others. The radical disjunct is shown by the remedy's prominence in two opposite descriptive rubrics: "Mind: desires to be carried," and "Mind: is averse to being carried."

The key theme of Bryonia, "everything worsens from movement," reflects well the contracted nature of Cold. During illness, patients seem to congeal themselves, turning away from others and preferring to remain physically still. They are prone to injuries resulting from continuous stop-and-go activity found in sports such as tennis. A general dryness of the mucous membranes and skin pertains to the congealed quality of Cold (think of the dryness of ice). The remedy state's pains are likely to crop up in response to the least exposure to the cold.

A typical Bryonia individual has dark hair and a dark complexion, with firm, fleshy fiber, is choleric, and has a bilious tendency. The remedy state has an affinity for individuals who overeat, especially meat, and have strong constitutions; it is a good fit with rich living. The diet of the Bryonia individual, rich in animal fats which are the primary source of arachidonic acid, is itself a prescription for arthritis. A variety of metabolic pathways transform arachidonic acid into prostaglandins (PGE2) as well as leukotrienes. It is debatable whether such dietary preferences predispose one to, or result from, the psoric mind-set. If one's preference is to be rid of Bryonia's characteristic swelling, tenseness, and knotted pain, then, in addition to taking the remedy, one should reduce one's reliance on animal fats and begin consuming some form of omega-3 and omega-6 fatty acids.

Rhus toxicodendron (Cold/Damp)

It is not unusual for Cold and Damp to be found in combination. Individuals in need of Rhus toxicodendron suffer from a "rusty-gate" syndrome in that they experience severe stiffness of the joints that is made worse by the cold or dampness and ameliorated by stretching and movement. Rhus toxicodendron people are restless, often itchy (the remedy is made from poison ivy), and drawn to a routine to the point of becoming superstitious. The mind-set pertaining to this challenge of being tightly contained within a structure from which one must also burst free creates a situation in which sudden movement is destabilizing. Contrary to Bryonia's association with tennis and the presence of a direct adversary, this remedy state is closely related to golf, in which the swing of the club demands exact repetition (the need to reach varying distances is met by switching clubs as opposed to altering the swing), and one's adversary is only oneself. Golfers are especially prone to back pain, often arthritic, for which Rhus tox is a key remedy.

Dulcamara (Cold/Damp)

Individuals in need of Dulcamara are prone to ailments from cold and wet weather or are subject to sudden climatic change. Their rheumatic pains involve coldness, and can be paralytic. The pains improve with physical movement, warmth, or the free flow of fluid secretions; that is, from a nasal discharge or episodic diarrhea which can ameliorate pain in this remedy state.

The anxiety of Dulcamara individuals relates to other persons such as friends, but mainly to family members. A patient's subconscious challenge—to seize control of the problems of those in her group with whom she overidentifies—is expressed in domineering behavior. Although her bossiness conveys an impression of anger, she would deny that this is the case. Her certitude of being correct is expressed as a fixed perspective that parallels the fixity of Damp Obstruction. A prescription of Dulcamara can mellow such individuals, while it greatly reduces their rheumatic pain.

Colchicum autumnale (Heat)

This remedy, made from autumn crocus, or meadow saffron, is of prime value in treating inflammatory gout, seen as a manifestation of the obstruction of Heat. As the ancient Chinese noted, however, Cold can transform into Heat. Underlying Colchicum's Heat lies the root cause of internal Cold, and it can either result from or produce interior food stagnation. In keeping with this logic, the remedy's materia medica reveals weaknesses that are conjoint with internal coldness as well as a tendency for an individual to collapse from loss of sleep and the ingestion of cold drinks and fatty foods.

Colchicum can also be studied from a dimensional perspective other than that of taste (the Earth Element). Individuals in need of this remedy are highly sensitive to the rudeness and misdeeds of others; moreover, the slightest touch from someone can send electric-like shocks throughout their body. These nervous symptoms, plus the indication that Colchicum individuals tend to be nauseous during the autumn, suggest that the remedy can also be viewed from the perspective of the dimension of sight (the Wood Element).

Colchicum's anxiety arises from "burning the candle at both ends." The remedy's radical disjunct describes the challenge of a person with a sensitive and sensuous nature who is drawn to overindulgence and then finds its effects unbearable. In clinical practice, the homeopath can reveal the need for Colchicum autumnale by observing that the patient not only is nauseated by food but also verbalizes a yearning for a simpler life.

Pulsatilla (Wind)

Also known in TCM as Moving Obstruction, Wind refers to pain in the joints that is widespread and moves from one area of the body to another. Pulsatilla's arthralgic pains and all its other symptoms manifest Wind because of their dramatic variance in quality, consistency, and location. The remedy's joint pains can include numbness, a distended sensation, heaviness, tearing pain, and swelling.

Pulsatilla is known primarily for its benefit to a woman who appears to have symptoms of hormonal imbalance. She may seem emotionally erratic, yet she basically feels vulnerable, even "forsaken." She is sympathetic, both in the sense of drawing another's sympathy toward herself and of having her own heart go out to anyone whom she perceives to be abandoned. In light of these symptoms, a woman in need of Pulsatilla has a tendency to cry easily.

What connects Pulsatilla's hormonally-driven symptoms with a sense of abandonment? As the menstrual cycle follows lunar rhythms and motions of the tides, a tidal metaphor may help us to understand why there is a connection. The anxiety of a woman in need of Pulsatilla relates to whether she feels loved. Whether or not she is loved, the challenge she faces is to master the tides, that is, to receive the comfort and consolation she needs.

Twice a day, during an interval known as slack tide, it is impossible to tell just by looking whether the ocean's tide is coming in or going out. The parallel metaphor is that of a woman's hormonal system, which, if disrupted as a result of disappointment or an experience of genuine abandonment, falls out of lunar rhythm. With hormonal instability substituted for her normal hormonal ebb and flow, the woman is then stuck at slack tide, her unmoored emotional state betrayed by the slack tide's uncertainty and randomness.

The physical symptoms associated with Pulsatilla further illuminate the remedy's radical disjunct. Despite her easy flow of tears, a Pulsatilla woman has a tendency to be congested, to inhibit a watery discharge. She may put her faith in the ease and naturalness of love, yet if she encounters the possibility of love she is provoked into feeling its opposite, a disbelief in and resistance to love.

A woman in need of Pulsatilla craves butter, pastries, and other comfort foods. Does her diet predispose her to Liver stagnation and associated weeping, or is it the other way around? In other words, does her belief that she is forsaken condemn her to make poor dietary choices and predispose her to wandering joint pain? As with many other conditions, the homeopath attempts to seek a suitable remedy without always knowing what in the illness is cause and what is effect.

TASTE DIMENSION ILLNESS: DIABETES

The body's fundamental metabolic challenge is how much energy it should liberate when it needs to respond to an emergency. Regarding the release of blood glucose, one speculative evolutionary theory argues that a climatic emergency, namely, the extremely cold temperatures that occurred at the onset of the Ice Age indirectly necessitated the liberation of short-term, but elevated energy levels.[7] Elevated blood glucose levels prevent a person's cells and tissues from forming ice crystals and thus help to keep him from freezing to death. This evolutionary theory suggests that the advent of the Ice Age may actually have prompted what is now known as juvenile diabetes to have survival value.

The question of what precisely constitutes a specific individual's emergency state varies hugely and defines his particular stresses. Before we examine the themes that underlie homeopathic remedies used in the treatment of diabetes, we will look first at the illness's challenges, that is, diabetes understood in terms of the metabolic burden. A condition whose defining symptom is a high level of blood glucose, diabetes is classically diagnosed as a failure of the body to properly metabolize carbohydrates. We suggest, however, that this may be largely inaccurate.

The prevalence of diabetes today is alarming. Data from the U.S. Centers for Disease Control and Prevention estimated that, in 2010, 25.8 million or 8.3% of the total U.S. population suffered from diabetes (18.8 million diagnosed, 7.0 million undiagnosed), and 26.9% of persons ages 65 years and older had diabetes. Moreover, in the period 2005 to 2008, over one-third of Americans ages 20 years or older were found by testing to have prediabetes.[8]

Diabetes is a disease that has become known variously as type 2 diabetes, insulin-resistant diabetes, insulin resistance, adult-onset diabetes, or more rarely, hyperinsulinemia. Gestational diabetes is ordinary diabetes contracted by a woman later in pregnancy whose metabolism is challenged by having to host a growing fetus.

Many of our degenerative diseases can be traced to a massive failure of the endocrine system, familiar to the physicians of the 1930s as insulin-resistant diabetes. Although diabetes is classically considered a failure of the body to properly metabolize carbohydrates, the disorder might better be described as a derangement of the blood-sugar control system caused by the burden of metabolizing inappropriate fats and oils and the consequent problems of cell-wall transport.

Obesity is considered a major risk factor for diabetes. Currently, over two-thirds of U.S. adults are either overweight or obese and over one-third are obese; in fact, from 1962 to 2006, the prevalence of obesity increased from about 13% to 35%.[9] Obesity is associated largely with a sedentary lifestyle and lack of exercise; a culturally endorsed and widespread consumption of empty calories and unhealthy fats; and the denaturing of foods which leaches out nutritionally vital minerals, such as chromium, that support metabolic function.

TASTE DIMENSION ILLNESS: TYPE I DIABETES

High blood glucose in type 1 diabetes—previously known as juvenile diabetes—results from insufficient insulin production by the pancreas, susceptibility to which may be inherited. The pancreatic underproduction of insulin and an inability to keep blood sugar within normal limits after eating may also be caused by a virus or by an autoimmune mechanism. As discussed in the chapter on the dimension of hearing, an inheritable susceptibility or congenital disorder may represent consolidation within Kidney Yang of a dysfunctional response that was introduced and reinforced within an individual's lineage ages ago. Thus, we recognize that type 1 diabetes exists on a continuum, developed largely from its hypoglycemic precursor condition, as opposed to and distinct from type 2 diabetes.

TASTE DIMENSION ILLNESS: TYPE 2 DIABETES

High glucose levels in type 2 diabetes result from ineffective insulin that fails to limit postprandial blood sugar levels to the normal range. Type 2 diabetes displays a radical disjunct in that elevated blood sugar levels are often preceded and accompanied by chronically elevated insulin levels. Hypoglycemia, or low blood sugar, can result from the same dietary and exercise deficiencies that give rise to diabetes. When the pancreas is stressed, insulin levels initially become elevated rather than deficient. If the pancreas continues to be overtaxed, it eventually tires of producing insulin, loses its ability to do so, and thus sets the stage for hyperglycemia, inadequate insulin levels, and diabetes. It helps to remember that steady, aerobic exercise provokes muscle-cell mitochondria, the powerhouse of the cell, to divide. With the excess power generated by surplus mitochondria, the pancreas is less prone to becoming overtaxed.

It is important to note that diabetes affects almost every cell in the seventy trillion or so cells of our body, each of which depends on the food we eat in order to acquire the raw materials that cells need for self-repair and maintenance. The ineffectiveness of insulin is caused not by the hormone itself, but by the body's cells being hindered in transporting glucose from the blood stream to the interior. When this occurs, glucose either remains in the blood stream, finds itself stored as body fat or glycogen, or is disposed of through urination.

METABOLIC PATHWAYS AND YIN DEFICIENCY

Whether a person with diabetes exhibits signs of excess (ruddiness, a thick coating on the tongue, constipation, strong personality) or—though less common in the West—of deficiency (frailty, tentativeness, weight-loss), one or more kinds of Yin deficiency are likely to be present. The primary diabetic Yin deficiency is that of Kidney Yin, which generally includes excessive thirst.

Insofar as the spleen is significantly responsible for metabolism, diabetes may be considered a metabolic disease. It is also true that the line between two disharmonies of fluids, the first pertaining to the spleen's transportation and transformation functions and the second to the kidneys' separation of the clean from the dirty, can be very thin. In TCM, crossing into Kidney's disharmony indicates that as the communication between fluid and vital heat control deteriorates, Yin and Yang come dangerously close to separating from one another. With the progression of the disease, the kidneys grow increasingly implicated in diabetes, which in TCM is known as Kidney Wasting Disease. In the chapter on the dimension of hearing, the kidney function is encountered in terms of its housing susceptibility to congenital diseases (as in type 1 diabetes) and its role in cell-membrane permeability.

The following pathway description provides a biomedical equivalent to the mucous and cell-membrane deterioration in TCM's depiction of how stress depletes Kidney Jing (essence): although not all the steps are as yet fully developed, it appears that when insulin binds to a cell-membrane receptor, it prompts a complex cascade of biochemical reactions inside the cell wherein a class of glucose transporters, known as GLUT 4 molecules, migrate from within the inside surface of the plasma cell membrane to eventually hook up with glucose molecules. In a process known as endocytosis, the glucose molecules are then transported into the interior of the cell where, in order to produce energy to power cellular activity, they are burned as fuel by the mitochondria. By thus transporting glucose out of the bloodstream into all of our body's cells, GLUT 4 transporters play a major role in lowering circulatory glucose.

Many of the molecules involved in these glucose- and insulin-mediated pathways are lipids, that is, they are fatty acids. A healthy plasma cell membrane, now known to be an active player in the glucose scenario, contains a complement of Cis-configured, omega-3, unsaturated fatty acids that renders the membrane relatively fluid and slippery. When a poor diet reduces the availability of fatty acids, substituted trans-fatty acids and short- and medium-chain saturated fatty acids make the cellular membrane stiffer, stickier, and more resistant to the glucose transport mechanism.

Thus, in the absence of sufficient Cis fatty acids in our diet, glucose remains elevated in the bloodstream. Elsewhere in the body, the pancreas secretes excess insulin, the liver manufactures fat from the excess sugar, the adipose cells store excess fat, the body goes into a high urinary mode, insufficient cellular energy is available for bodily activity, and the entire endocrine system is disharmonized. Eventually pancreatic failure occurs, body weight plummets, and a diabetic crisis is precipitated.

It is important to remember that not all fats and oils are created equal. Many saturated oils and fats are highly beneficial, while many unsaturated oils are not. The health distinction is not really between saturated and unsaturated, as the fats and oils industry would have us believe, but between the consequences of consuming oils that are natural, such as vegetable, flax, fish, and coconut oils, and those that are engineered, such as soy, cottonseed, and rape seed oils.

TASTE DIMENSION ILLNESS: DIABETES
HOMEOPATHIC REMEDIES

Dozens of remedies may be of use in diabetic conditions. Of these, four have been selected because of their special affinity for diabetes and for their ability to illustrate core themes pertaining to the dimension of taste; a fifth, Syzygium jambolanum, has been chosen for its specific action in reducing blood sugar.

Helonias-Chamaelirium: "A Woman's Work Is Never Done"

Also known as Veratrum luteum, or false unicorn root, Helonias is an excellent remedy for the initial stage of diabetes insipidus when a sensation of weakness first makes itself known. Its use is historically indicated primarily for women challenged by too many physical demands. These women become exhausted from too many pregnancies or by hard labor, or they may grow enfeebled from producing insufficient blood to make up for blood lost in menstruation. Perhaps not surprisingly, given what we know about muscular tone in relation to the balance of pancreatic hormones, Helonias is indicated for individuals who are worn out, not only by actual strain, but also by excesses of luxury or indolence.

The homeopathic materia medica describes a clinical picture consistent with deficiency of either Kidney Yin or Kidney Yang (both can be deficient). Among women, the remedy's symptoms may include a sense of weightiness of one's womb, excessive awareness of the womb itself, severe lower backache, radiating chill, but also heat flushes.

The remedy's telling mental and emotional feature, that a woman feels better when she is mentally busy, directs us to Helonias's central anxiety and radical disjunct: weakness and the loss of the capacity to produce blood, symptoms that should confirm that her work is done, instead prove the reverse, that her work is in fact not done. Perhaps a means may be found other than Helonias to dispel the delusion that to remain vital, a woman must remain physically productive.

Argentum nitricum

Argentum nitricum is another remedy that is useful in the early stages of diabetes. Derived from silver nitrate, its keynote symptoms include an extreme craving for sugar, frequently conjoint with heightened anxiety after eating sugar. The disharmonious relationship with sugar may either stem from or reflect carnality.

Another characteristic feature is that individuals needing the remedy crave both sugar and salt. The sugar-craving individual is suggestible and impulsive, while the salt-craving person exhibits a contractive quality (salt causes water to be contained within cells) and is recalcitrant when presented with reasonable objectives.

Linked together, the sugar and salt aspects create an unusual picture: The Argentum nitricum individual is herky-jerky, physically awkward, and quirky. Prone to terrible anticipatory anxiety, he is likely to perceive a pending examination or performance as a major ordeal. In his dread he behaves as if future demands are immediately at hand. One such patient informed me that she always begins packing for a trip months ahead of time. Physical symptoms include urinary insecurity, belching and abdominal discomfort, chronic hoarseness, trembling, and debility.

Argentum nitricum's radical disjunct relates to the everyday assessment of surrounding hazards. An individual who is not in this remedy state unconsciously calculates how surrounding or upcoming challenges will forward his well-being. The inner safety engineer of the Argentum nitricum individual, however, responds with panic to this experience. Perhaps a means other than Argentum nitricum can be found to dispel the inner safety engineer's exaggerated response.

Saccharum officinale: "Sweetness and Blight"

The domain of the dimension of taste obviously includes flavor. Of the five flavors, according to TCM sweetness is the flavor specifically associated with Earth and metabolism. Also known as cane sugar or white sugar, Saccharum is an old, but in many ways timely, remedy that is relevant because rather than being digested in the mouth or stomach, sugar goes straight to the large intestine and moves quickly into the blood stream. A rapid rise in blood-sugar levels promotes what is in effect a temporary diabetic state.

Saccharum is of great value in the treatment not only of diabetes but of hyperactivity, obesity, a wide range of addictive disorders, mouth ulcers, suppressed immune response, malnutrition, mineral and vitamin deficiency, and bowel and stomach disorders. The anxiety displayed by a Saccharum individual stems from having a lack of sufficient power to meet an emergency. Unfortunately, the quick-fix sugar solution to an emergency is deceiving, as sugar is both an antiseptic and a preservative, killing anything in its immediate vicinity.

White sugar promotes the power that comes with weight gain (a false substantiality) while it decays living tissue. As Melissa Assilem points out in *The Mad Hatter's Tea Party*,[10] Saccharum's core situation relates to an experience common in childhood, that of being bribed with candy to suppress legitimate anger. Thus Saccharum's radical disjunct is laid bare: cheaply bought or falsely acquired, regenerative energy brings forth its polar opposite, decomposition.

Kreosotum

The name "Kreosotum" derives from the Greek meaning "flesh preserver." Also known as beechwood creosote and made from liquid pitch oil, this remedy, like sugar, both preserves and destroys flesh. Because it addresses advanced pathology, Kreosotum pertains as much to the dimensions of sight and hearing as to taste; but as the remedy's domain resembles that of Saccharum, albeit with a deeper and more extensive pathology, it is described here.

The remedy state features irritability, fear, premature decaying of the teeth, coldness of the extremities, hemorrhaging, and burning pain. Kreosotum, in relation to diabetes, is often described as being of use in situations in which the trophic nervous system is depressed, stagnating growth. The patient experiences a general heaviness with drowsiness; a depression of spirits; a confused and dull feeling in the head; dim-sightedness; a flat, bitter taste; an appetite with a sensation of fullness; intermittent, hard, dry stools; frequent and copious emissions of hot, clear urine; a bruised sensation in the chest and all along the back; physical exhaustion, which is worse after rest; and a great itching of the genitals during and after micturation.

In TCM terms, these symptoms suggest a diagnosis of exhaustion of Kidney Yang, combined with Liver Fire. Robin Logan, whose remarks are reprinted in Vermeulin's *Prisma* discussion of Kreosotum,[11] describes a mental and emotional state arising from or reflecting situations requiring a commitment to self-preservation. If a means other than Kreosotum could effectively dispel the delusional aspect of this commitment to self-preservation, it would be heavy therapy indeed.

Syzygium jambolanum

Syzygium jambolanum is made from the fruit of the tree called the jambul, which is indigenous to the South Asian and Australian regions. Syzygium in low-potency doses is highly effective in lowering blood sugar. Numerous reports from India indicate that when taken at appropriate intervals (which may require some trial and error) it is found to both significantly palliate diabetes mellitus and, on occasion, perform curatively. Because we are unacquainted with its mental and emotional features, Syzygium lingers in a unique category for the purposes of our characteristic analysis; it is therefore currently not possible to describe the remedy's radical disjunct and place it within a specific sense dimension.

TASTE DIMENSION ILLNESS: CHRONIC FATIGUE SYNDROME

As described in the chapter on the dimension of sight, the depletion of energy and the associated gastrointestinal dysfunction usually manifest because of a poor resolution of the conflict between creativity and chaos (which can translate as anger stagnating the Liver). To the extent to which this is not the case, however, chronic fatigue and its associated gastrointestinal ailments are for the most part a failing governed by the dimension of taste, and result from a poor resolution of taste's core issue, anxiety versus challenge.

The concept that chronic fatigue has a biological basis in mitochondrial disorders is rapidly gaining credence. Although now considered to be the most prevalent of all metabolic diseases, mitochondrial disorders were once thought to be relatively rare. Diseases with dysfunctional mitochondrial traits include the syndrome of mitochondrial encephalomyopathy, lactic acidosis, and stroke-like episodes (MELAS); myoclonic epilepsy with ragged-red fibers (MERRF); and Leber's hereditary optic neuropathy (LHON).

TASTE DIMENSION ILLNESSES: MITOCHONDRIAL DISORDERS
NUTRITIONAL SUPPLEMENTS

Adopting a biometabolic strategy to address metabolic dysfunction is only logical. Nutritional supplements such as the following show evidence of being able to help combat and protect against mitochondrial decay:

- *Glutathione* plays a key role in protecting the mitochondria's inner membrane and the mitochondrial DNA itself from oxidative damage.

- *N-acetyl cysteine* is a natural precursor of glutathione.

- *B-Complex vitamins* supply levels of B-vitamins in excess of required dosage. They strengthen coenzyme binding to oxidant-damaged enzymes. As a result, enzymatic activity against aging and oxidant damage is increased.

- *Nicotinamide adenine dinucleotide (NADH)* is a coenzyme that is the biochemical active form of niacin (vitamin B-3). It is present in all living cells and stimulates adenosine triphosphate (ATP) production.

- *Acetyl L-carnitine* serves as a precursor for acetyl CoA, the start of the citric acid cycle.

- *Lipoic acid* scavenges free radicals and regenerates other antioxidants.

- *Adenosine triphosphate (ATP)* may provide a shortcut to the elevation of ATP levels in the cells as it can be taken orally and converted into adenosine monophosphate (AMP) and adenosine diphosphate (ADP).

- *Coenzyme Q10 (CoQ10)* is a key player in the mitochondrial electron transport chain. *Idebenone* is a synthetic analog (variation) of CoQ10.

• ***Deprenyl***, used extensively in Europe since 1970, is an antiaging drug that works by inhibiting an enzyme that breaks down dopamine, thereby elevating dopamine levels in the brain and in the central nervous system.

TASTE DIMENSION ILLNESSES: MITOCHONDRIAL DISORDERS
HOMEOPATHIC REMEDIES

As with acupuncture, in which numerous treatment strategies may apply, a virtually limitless number of homeopathic remedies are of potential use in addressing a mitochondrial syndrome. From among this profusion, three carbon-based remedies have been chosen for analysis. The materia medica of each of these remedies reflects the adverse affect mitochondrial dysfunction can exert on living tissue as well as the specific mental/emotional dynamic likely to predispose a patient to mitochondrial failure.

Carbo animalis

Carbo animalis, a remedy made from animal charcoal, is of use in states involving physical burnout. Individuals in need of Carbo animalis lack vital heat; are prone to slow, painfully developing, and sometimes cancerous, conditions; have poor circulation; and are rigid. Their energy is stagnant and dry, like an old piece of charred leather the remedy is made from.

Carbo animalis individuals are also prone to nostalgia, homesickness, and a longing for the past, all of which reflects an anxiety regarding the aging process and an unconscious desire to turn back time. Their rigid determination to keep things as they are represents an unmet challenge to their ability to expend metabolic energy efficiently. The remedy's radical disjunct is manifested as resistance to aging only serves to hasten aging. A patient of mine, an adolescent girl holding fundamentalist religious values not espoused within her family, complained that her hands often felt as though they belonged to an old, arthritic woman. A dose of Carbo animalis eliminated this delusion within days.

Carbo vegetabilis

Carbo vegetabilis, a remedy made from vegetable charcoal, is similar to carbo animalis in its use in burned-out states. Like Carbo animalis, its materia medica is a portrait of stagnation, low energy, fearfulness, and apathy that appears to result from an exhausting disease or an abusive lifestyle. Carbo vegetablilis, although a slow-acting remedy, is frequently an excellent resource in chronic fatigue syndrome. The Carbo vegetabilis individual has tremendous difficulty in rousing herself in order to do anything. She has a paradoxical symptom, which reveals the remedy's radical disjunct: despite feeling chilled, she craves exposure to a cool breeze. Picture an allegory of a faintly glowing ember, fearful of the blaze of the fireplace, but filled with anxiety to conserve its vital warmth, that is, not to be blown out. Its challenge is to keep itself glowing, in order to have sufficient oxygen to fuel its metabolic furnace.

Graphites

An individual in need of Graphites, or mineral carbon, lacks sensitivity to impressions, is chilly, dull, and irresolute. Her attraction is to basic earth pleasures such as gardening. She is likely to be an untidy dresser.

The remedy state Graphites is the opposite of Phosphorus, which is used in cases of anxiety disorder and is characterized by a spark of creative energy and an excess of in-touchness. A Graphites patient, in contrast, despairs that she can ever touch the source of creation, and she remains overly concerned with the organic disintegration that eventually overtakes all living things. When confronted with even trifling issues, she crumbles like the tip of a lead pencil when it is pressed down too hard.

The principal sphere of pathology in Graphites is the skin, which is prone to becoming thick, dry, and fissured. In TCM, within the sense dimension of taste, we are likely to diagnose a deficiency of Spleen blood that fails to nourish the skin.[12]

Graphites represents a picture of thwarted or stunted creativity, a subconscious notion that given different conditions, "I could have been a carbon form with a better organized crystal structure—a diamond perhaps." Graphites' radical disjunct relates to the fact that carbon is the great connector in organic life forms: faced with a personal crisis, the Graphites' patient overconnects materially, thus hastening material decomposition. In the process she grows so thickened materially that eventually even cellular mitochondria are discouraged. Whether it reflects or predisposes mitochondrial dysfunction, the delusion of being dense must be overcome, perhaps by using substances other than Graphites.

TASTE DIMENSION ILLNESS:
GASTROESOPHAGEAL REFLUX DISEASE (GERD)

In TCM, gastroesophageal reflux disease (GERD) is referred to as Rebellious Stomach Qi. Normally when one eats or drinks, the lower esophageal sphincter (LES), the muscle at the bottom of the tube known as the esophagus, closes off. This enables foods and liquids to remain sequestered in the stomach. TCM describes this as the downward pull of Stomach Qi. If the reverse occurs, stomach acid touches the lining of the esophagus. A burning sensation in the chest or throat, familiar to many of us as heartburn, then results. When the flow of this fluid extends to the back of the mouth it is called acid indigestion, acid reflux, or heartburn. Occasional heartburn is not uncommon, but heartburn occurring more than twice weekly may be considered to be the chronic condition, gastroesophageal reflux disease. Undealt with, it can eventually lead to increasingly serious health problems.

GERD indicates the existence of excessive anxiety within the dimension of taste, which causes digestion to be experienced as an overly formidable challenge. Additional symptoms indicative of GERD include some of the following:

- Chest pain
- Hoarseness on waking
- Difficulty with swallowing, or a choking sensation
- A sensation of food being lodged in the throat
- The eructation and regurgitation of food
- A persistent dry cough
- Halitosis

In biomechanical terms, GERD may result when the esophagus's normal defenses may be inadequate relative to the acid content of the stomach; when the contents of the stomach may themselves be overly acidic; or when food fails to clear out of the esophagus swiftly enough. As we know, however, illness does not occur randomly. As health caregivers we must ask: What emotional states might predispose any of these events to happen consistently and cause an individual to develop GERD?

TASTE DIMENSION ILLNESS:
GASTROESOPHAGEAL REFLUX DISEASE (GERD)
NUTRITIONAL STRATEGIES

By following the nutritional strategies listed below, a patient may help to minimize the symptoms of GERD:

- Avoid alcohol and spicy, fatty, or acidic foods
- Eat smaller meals
- Don't eat close to bedtime
- Lose weight if you are obese
- Wear loose-fitting clothes

TASTE DIMENSION ILLNESS:
GASTROESOPHAGEAL REFLUX DISEASE (GERD)
HOMEOPATHIC REMEDIES

A vast number of homeopathic remedies may be called into play with regard to GERD. GERD reflects the extensive morbidity and excessive anxiety that can be represented within the dimension of taste, combined with a plethora of symptoms relating to anxiety within the materia medica of the mind. While homeopathy provides a wealth of treatment possibilities, an overabundance of choices in regard to redressing GERD can also overwhelm the health care practitioner. The practitioner must therefore pay close attention to associated modalities—situations that improve or worsen the symptoms—in selecting a remedy in materia medica within extensive rubrics such as stomach, eructations–general; or stomach, eructations–water brash; or stomach–heartburn. It is also important to make note of any unusual features the patient reports.

After completing a careful winnowing of the list of possible remedies, the practitioner is required to make a rigorous differentiation among the remaining remedies. The practitioner must then seek to match key issues underlying the patient's anxiety with the anxiety theme underlying the short-listed remedy. Constitutional homeopaths are already aware that whether it presents as GERD or as another condition, each case must be undertaken thoroughly, completely, and in its totality. Otherwise key clues leading to the most accurate remedy can be missed.

THE TASTE DIMENSION: PERSONAL THERAPEUTIC PRACTICES AND MASTERS OF EXPRESSION

In addition to options in acupuncture, homeopathy, and biomedicine, a range of therapeutic practices can help promote health within the sense dimension of taste. **Table 1** lists several of these practices.

A number of masters throughout history have strongly expressed the positive and negative poles of the sense dimension of taste. **Table 2** on the following page lists several of these masters who exemplified one or the other side of the challenge-anxiety axis, the core issue of the dimension of taste.

Table 1. Taste Dimension: Health-promoting Practices

Chew and taste food thoroughly	**Exercise regularly**
Cook with care and artistry	**Experience hunger and satiety**
Eat a nutritious, varied diet	**Honor the feminine**
Use local and seasonal foods	**Savor wisdom and knowledge**
Nurture the mother of taste, *Touch*: "Maintain a regular spiritual practice"	**Identify, evaluate, and accept challenges**

Table 2. Examples of Masters of the Sense Dimension of Taste

NEGATIVE POLE: ANXIETY	POSITIVE POLE: CHALLENGE
Franz Kafka	Arthur Schopenhauer
Woody Allen	Ayn Rand
	Karl Marx
	Charles Darwin (survival of the fittest)
	Spiritual sources evoking Shekina (DivinePresence), Mary, Shakti, Isis, other aspects of the Goddess

CHAPTER FIVE

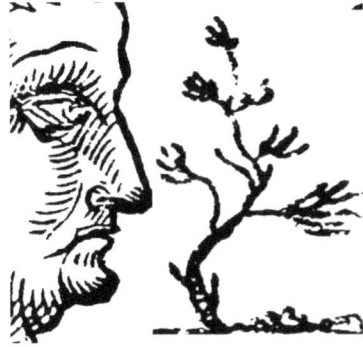

THE DIMENSION OF SMELL

THE SENSE DIMENSION OF SMELL

PHASE	METAL
ORGAN	LUNG
CORE ISSUE	CENTEREDNESS-DISORIENTATION

Smell is the chemical sense that enables us to detect signs and signals at a distance. Smell orients us with respect to environmental conditions, such as in the smell of fire and of rain. Scent markings inform us of the presence of various animals. We locate plants by their fragrances, and then imitate them with perfumes. Of all species, perhaps the most striking example of the orienting power of smell is the salmon: It depends primarily on smell to guide it on the long journey back to its stream of origin to spawn.

By smell we identify and attract mates, communicate our emotional state, advertise the genotype of our immune system, signal illness, and bond with our kin. Each person emits an individual smell signature, one that is transiently influenced by the smell of foods he eats. Smell is also a major component of flavor, contributing to the distinction between edible and inedible foods. We are not conscious of all the smells we register and react to, and sometimes we are led by the nose.

Smell occurs primarily through receptors in the nose, which send signals processed by the brain. New genetic research suggests that not odor receptors, but the nervous system's wiring actually determines how odors are defined.[1]

Smells are powerfully and durably linked with memory and emotion, and they can obliterate time: whiffing the odor of a cigar recreates childhood visits with a favorite uncle. But smell also happens on imperceptible levels. For example, sperm have chemoreceptors that orient them by smell to locate an egg.

The sense of smell is less acute in humans than it is in mammals. Part of the human sense of smell may have been displaced by increased acuity of vision and touch. With aging, humans lose some ability to smell; the significant majority of octogenarians have chronic dysfunctions of smell. In those who have Alzheimer's disease, the sense of smell declines markedly early in the course of the disease.

THE LUNGS IN TRADITIONAL CHINESE MEDICINE

The Lungs in TCM are conceived of as the ruler of the Qi, which they help to form and then distribute downwards throughout the body. The Lungs govern respiration, bringing in pure Qi and expelling impure Qi. The Lungs receive nutritive fluids from the Spleen, and Lung Qi moves and balances these fluids. As the ruler of the body's exterior, the Lungs contribute not only to the condition of the skin, but to the defensive energy that protects the body from disease. Thus, in biomedical terms, the lungs provide immune system functions. The Lungs and their paired organ, Large Intestine, belong to the Phase of Metal, which is associated with the autumn, and with crying and grief.

The Lungs are said to house the Po, or Corporeal Soul. In TCM the Po is the equivalent of our bodily animal spirit. This animating presence lives and dies with the body, and is sustained with us through breathing. All breathing creatures have a Corporeal Soul, a mark of brotherhood among animal life forms.

The signs and symptoms of Lung disorders in TCM include acute and chronic respiratory disorders, inflammation of the nose or throat, coughing, excessive phlegm, loss of voice, spontaneous sweating, allergies to airborne substances, and dry skin. Disorders of the colon (e.g., constipation, irritable bowel syndrome) may be included because of the energetic link with the Lungs' paired organ, Large Intestine. Ménière's disease, discussed within the context of the dimension of hearing in Chapter 6, includes a disorientation symptom, namely vertigo, that not surprisingly also reflects the pathology of the Lungs: Phlegm and dampness obstruct the Middle Burner, part of one of the six Yang organs in the body, and suppress the Qi of respiration (also known as the Cleansing Yang Qi) that rises to the eyes, ears, nose, and mouth in order to maintain the clarity of the senses.

Respiration orients us to the past and the future. We take our first breath at birth, an inhalation of air and of the future before us. In death, a conclusive exhalation releases us from connection to past experience. In between birth and death, at an average of sixteen times a minute, we repeat this same activity which involves embracing the future and releasing ourselves from the past. The Qi gong master believes that by mastering inward breath, allowing it to fully extend downwards, into the Cinnabar Field[2] below the navel and within the abdomen (which the Chinese refer to as the dantien), a kind of immortality is achieved. This does not mean he cannot die, but rather that, having achieved mastery over all possibilities, he no longer worries about the future. The Qi gong master knows that mastering the extended, exhaled breath bodes freedom from attachment to the fleeting past and unencumbered participation in the life-energy sparkling amid the emptiness of the universe. Ordinary language also reflects an inherent linkage of inhalation and freedom within the context of independence. Thus the word inspiration denotes both the inhaled breath and receptiveness to astonishing ideas.

To follow the Tao means to seek mastery of both the inward and outward breath and therefore of the present, the future, and the past. It was often said in ancient times that to achieve the Tao matters less than setting out in the general direction of the Tao. This option and its attendant health benefits lie completely within the reach of ordinary people, not only Qi gong masters.

SMELL DIMENSION CORE ISSUE: THE CENTEREDNESS-DISORIENTATION AXIS

In the course of animal evolution, physiologic respiration moved from exterior surfaces to inside the body. Single-celled creatures exchange gases through cell-wall surfaces; frogs conduct respiration through their moist skins. As an animal's size increases, the surface area of the skin becomes insufficient to support the greater requirements of gas exchange. The lungs in an adult human provide about 70 square meters of total surface area. Meeting these higher demands on physiologic respiration has drawn the location of breathing inward to the body's center.

There is also a connection between our psychological sense of centeredness and the locus of breathing. In panic attacks, breathing becomes rapid and shallow; in fact, this pattern of breathing may bring on a sense of panic. In panic we experience a loss of grounding, a psychological decentering in which rational control is wrested away by signals from the reptilian brain. Some individuals assert control over panic attacks and regain their centeredness by focusing on deep abdominal breathing.

CENTEREDNESS

To be centered or oriented means to be aware of one's self in one's surroundings. This aspect of centeredness or orientation may be spatial, environmental, cultural, social, or spiritual. There is also a temporal aspect to orientation, an awareness of the present moment tempered by relevant history and future possibilities.

Orientation takes a decidedly interior turn with respect to breathing. With every breath, we define our center by the depth of our relationship with the plenum of air, to which all other beings are simultaneously attached. The presence and penetration of the aromatic air orients us not only to all it conveys, but to our own central core. In a very real sense, each inhalation brings our future, while each exhalation removes our past. Thus, mastery of breathing orients us in the present with respect to past and future. No wonder that so many meditative practices emphasize attending to the breath, and that breath and spirit share the same linguistic root in so many languages. Breathing constitutes the foundation of centeredness.

DISORIENTATION

Disorientation is the opposing pole to centeredness on this axis. Our compass may become skewed or utterly lost, leaving us unable to locate or balance self-interest and communal interest. We may fall into temporal distortions, grieving, and unable to part with a preferred past, or frozen in terror by a traumatic event from years long ago. Lacking resolution and inspiration, we limp through life like one wounded. This ingrained disorientation then manifests through symptoms of chronic illness.

SMELL DIMENSION: CHRONIC ILLNESSES

Confirmation of how central orientation and direction is to the sense of smell comes from the field of organic chemistry. Scientists in the fragrance industry have discovered that the nose assigns different odors to chemicals whose otherwise identical molecular structures are mirror images of one another. In other words, and to the subtlest degree imaginable, the nose knows its right from its left.[3]

SMELL DIMENSION ILLNESS: ALLERGIES

Why do we suffer allergies to grass, tree pollens, cat dander, dust mites, and mold spore, or why is such a lethal reaction caused in some people after eating peanuts or shrimps? As an inherent part of the immune system, allergic reactions at some point in our evolution likely served an important purpose. For example, as suggested in the chapter on touch, an apparently random sensitivity to gluten underlying celiac disease may have protected society at large by predisposing certain individuals to survive outbreaks of ergotism. Of course, like the anaphylactic shock from eating peanuts, certain allergies can present problems too severe to discount. Otherwise, to the extent to which annoying seasonal sneezing or itching of the eyes can be withstood, a partnering approach to allergies is preferred to a reliance on medication that suppresses the immune system.

SMELL DIMENSION ILLNESS: ALLERGIES
HOMEOPATHIC REMEDY

Kali carbonicum

Allergies can result when disorientation triumphs over centeredness. To illustrate, we draw on an example of analysis and treatment with a homeopathic remedy. The homeopathic remedy Kali carbonicum effectively treats allergies in an individual whose personality type hinges on the centeredness versus disorientation conundrum. The black-and-white Kali carbonicum personality adheres closely to a moral code that he expects others to also follow, and holds loyalty and honesty at a premium. Significantly, the Kali carbonicum individual is both mentally rigid and unusually sensitive to dampness.

An inability to be subtle and to detect subtle amounts of moisture in the nasal mucosa express one and the same issue. The olfactory apparatus is nestled in the nasal mucosa. A Kali carbonicum individual reflects a parallel relationship between an issue of directionality ("I can go only to the right or the left, not in-between") and the mucosa's inability or unwillingness to process moisture. In a person who is insensitive to Kali carbonicum, moisture is processed away by the nasal mucosa just as quickly as its presence is detected. In someone sensitive to Kali carbonicum, however, moisture accumulating in the nasal mucosa is not detected until there is far too much of it, at which point, an overreaction to moisture in the guise of an allergy attack erupts.

SMELL DIMENSION ILLNESSES:
ASTHMA AND PANIC DISORDER

Gasping, a sharp intake of breath, is a common respiratory response to shock. A panic attack, serial gasping (not panting), manifests as a rapid and seemingly uncontrollable intake of breath. The brain overoxygenates, causing nervous excitement and fear to spiral further.

Individuals suffering from panic attacks temporarily suffer a delusion that they are sure to die soon. In response to a past experience of shock or exhaustion, a panicking individual, in fact, inhales too much of the future and loses the current connection with the source of his breath. Try gasping serially for a few moments while also looking in a mirror; it is unlikely you can do so without raising your shoulders, constricting your lungs, and appearing very anxious.

Wheezing is the diametrical opposite of gasping. Its pattern of asthmatic respiration may express overattachment to an emotionally suppressive past (and a consequent loss of connection to the source of the breath). Though desperate to exhale his past into oblivion, the wheezing asthmatic individual creates a shortage of oxygen. In a spiraling pattern, an increasing deficit of oxygen heightens anxiety and desperation, thereby further accelerating a stimulus to wheeze. Persons with asthma who wheeze often have had a childhood in which the natural expression of emotion had been systematically suppressed—an experience not unlike suffocation. Wheezing, a form of self-suffocation, subconsciously grants the patient with asthma permission to dramatize the pain of emotional suppression while simultaneously trying to cast off its suffocating consequences.

Frequent asthmatic episodes can produce a cascade in which a chronic inflammatory response and mucous buildup in the airways promote secondary breathing problems and additional anxiety. According to TCM, asthma is always rooted in misdirection, in the failure of the Lung Qi to descend. A partnering with the asthmatic condition so as to redress it now suggests itself: in order to encourage the Qi to descend, a person with asthma must learn to embrace, rather than fear, his omens.

Dreaded or not, future moments do not overwhelm centered individuals. Rather, each moment is calmly encountered in its own good time. Once centering is mastered, respiratory symptoms decrease in severity and frequency, or else vanish entirely, without recourse to drugs. Relaxation techniques, meditation, and yoga practices that embrace breathing exercises abound. Simple techniques promoting the descending movement of Lung Qi and reconnection with the source of the breath can be quickly learned and easily practiced. We are thus directed to achieve mastery of the past, the present, and the future.

SMELL DIMENSION ILLNESSES: HOARSENESS AND LOSS OF VOICE

Song and speech are created by means of the breath propelling a sound wave shaped within the larynx and cavities of the head. The loss or distortion of the voice occurs when one's connection to the source of the breath is broken. The head and larynx are, in effect, instruments that must be neither overly moist nor overly dry so as to produce a clear and pleasing sound. If the mucous membranes within the head are clogged, a nasal whine is produced.[4] Within the larynx, this relates to the Yin (natural moisture) of the Lungs, which, should they become deficient, dry out the larynx, causing hoarseness and loss of the voice.

When laryngitis occurs suddenly and not as a result of abuse of the voice, the possibility of an emotional cause has to be considered. TCM theory holds, in fact, that excessive worry dries out the body's fluids. Clinical homeopathic experience indicates that women are more inclined than men are to be subject to an emotional loss of the voice, a condition treated with great effectiveness with Ignatia. This homeopathic remedy is appropriate in situations in which a shocking grief has suddenly turned a woman's life upside down, producing, not only a loss of the voice, but disorientation and frequently depression as well.

SMELL DIMENSION ILLNESSES:
SKIN AILMENTS: PSORIASIS, ECZEMA, ACNE

Although amphibians, reptiles, and mammals have lungs housed within their chest cavities, the lungs are specialized organs that did not appear on the scene until the evolution of the lungfish. Yet, older and more primitive organisms, even those consisting of only a single cell, also respire. They do so by means of an exchange of gases that occurs through the cell membrane of the skin. Even without the benefit of microscopes, TCM, which demonstrates that acupuncture points located along the Lung meridian are indicated in the treatment of most skin conditions, preserves this biological truth. Similarly, TCM describes the numerous wrinkles and extraordinary creases found in the faces of long-time smokers in terms of the depletion of Lung Yin (natural moisture).

Like frogs, in whose always-moist skin some exchange of gases necessarily occurs, we, through skin rashes and eruptions, attempt to vent internal toxins. Skin rashes and eruptions may also express a deficiency in our ability to vent a pernicious entity known in TCM as Damp Heat. We find echoes of outer membrane gas exchanges in TCM's Qi gong vital energy exercises. Here, a vestigial (or literal) ability to respire through the skin is invoked by the Qi gong instructor's directive that the practitioner visualize herself breathing through every pore in her body.

Dozens of homeopathic remedies may be used to assist the body in clearing it of internal heat and toxicity. Of these, the most frequently used is undoubtedly Sulphur.

SMELL DIMENSION ILLNESSES:
LARGE INTESTINE AILMENTS:
CONSTIPATION AND IRRITABLE BOWEL SYNDROME (IBS)

Like the skin, the intestines are an interface surface that functions as a protective barrier. The intestines sequester bacteria-laden digestive matter from the rest of the abdominal cavity. The esophageal-intestinal tract is a continuous tube, extending from the mouth to the rectum. In addition to food, air and other gases enter this tract. Although oxygen does not undergo oxidation within the gut, gas exchanges and gas production from the intestinal flora do occur. The expulsion of these gases from the tract's terminus thus qualifies the esophageal-intestinal tract, in a metaphorical sense at least, as a secondary site of respiration. In its pairing of the two organs in theory, TCM recognizes the overlapping function of the lungs and large intestine viscera.

Acupuncture Points as Treatment

The acupuncture meridians pertaining to the Lungs and the Large Intestine are found positioned side by side on the upper limbs. The key to treating patients who experience symptoms of the Lung and the Large Intestine simultaneously, as well as symptoms of skin conditions, is an acupuncture point (Lung 7), located on the wrist where the two meridians intersect. Another acupuncture point, renowned for its effectiveness in the treatment of skin disorders, is a Large Intestine point located on the outer elbow (Large Intestine 11). Stimulation of an acupuncture point found on the lower leg (Stomach 40) helps the body process excessive mucous, whether it is lodged in the lungs or in the intestines.

SMELL DIMENSION ILLNESSES:
LARGE INTESTINE AILMENTS:
CONSTIPATION AND IRRITABLE BOWEL SYNDROME (IBS)
HOMEOPATHIC REMEDY

Natrum sulphuricum

Healthful bowel activity can be understood as a steady downward and outward movement. According to TCM, dampness, mucous, and excessive dryness afflict the airways and intestines in a similar fashion: Dampness and mucous can cause diarrhea, as well as an uncontrolled urge to move the bowels; dryness produces constipation. The obstruction and dysfunction of the intestines may be construed to be a disordered digestive exhalation. Conversely, for the intestines, the airways, and mental functioning, the feeling of being clear corresponds with a state of health.

Because the diagnosis of irritable bowel syndrome includes a vast number of symptoms, dozens of homeopathic remedies are of potential use. One in particular is noted for its thematic aptness: Natrum sulphuricum, also known as sodium sulfate, or Glauber's salt. Its natrum component addresses grief (disorientation-in-time); its sulphurous component relates to the presence of internal Heat. Natrum sulphuricum's famous keynote, "better after a bowel movement," implies a psychologically driven need to feel clear.

SMELL DIMENSION ILLNESSES: MENTAL DISORDERS

The emotion that TCM designates as specific to the viscera of the Lungs is sad-ness, or grief. The fact that in sobbing the entire chest heaves reminds us of this. It is not unusual to become sad when we look at the falling leaves of autumn, when we are most reminded of our mortality—the season which TCM associates with the dimension of smell.

After a tragedy or loss, a mysterious process of self-regulation enables the be-reaved to eventually attain distance from the loss. If prolonged or excessive pres-sure is brought to bear on a person's particular sensibility, this process can even be short-circuited. It is a fallacy to assume that each of us is saddened by exactly the same experiences, or to the same degree or length of time. Our constitution and its individual hot-button wiring account for profound differences in reactions. To the extent that it affects the particular individual, insufficiently processed grief stresses the Lungs, and thereby may also play a role in predisposing lung and breast cancer.

SMELL DIMENSION ILLNESS:
SEASONAL AFFECTIVE DISORDER (SAD)

Although a case can be made that depression arising from the deprivation of sunlight, namely, seasonal affective disorder (SAD), is rooted in the dimen-sion of sight, I interpret SAD as expressing disorientation, which pertains primar-ily to the dimension of smell. The shortening of daylight hours in wintertime may cause many of us to become blue, but the distress of the SAD individual can be overwhelming. Listless and depressed, he droops much like a plant that fails to orient itself adequately to the sun.

Sunlight and water are key components of a respiration process known as pho-tosynthesis, by which plants manufacture their own nutrients. It is fair to say that plants deprived of sunlight fear imminent starvation. Light-starved SAD individu-als suffer the unbalancing of their master gland of homeostasis, the hypothalamus. As a result, regulation of numerous vital functions becomes problematic.

The hypothalamus's main function is maintenance of our body's status quo, the grounding of our physical existence in the present moment. The hypothala-mus is responsible for creating and sustaining set points for our blood pressure and skin temperature. It determines what level of toxicity our blood can carry or our brain tissue can be exposed to before detoxification by expulsive vomiting is required. Because the limbic and olfactory systems project to the hypothalamus, the gland plays a major role in regulating hunger and sexual desire. In regulating our circadian rhythms and synchronizing them with daylight and darkness, the hypothalamus also sets our sleep patterns.

We can rebalance the hypothalamus and overcome SAD by inhaling additional sunlight through the pores. By combining maximal outdoor activity with periodic, indoor exposure to full-spectrum lighting similar to sunlight, we help our body recover its physical bearings. Inhalation of sunlight orients our body to the demands of the present moment.

SMELL DIMENSION ILLNESS: SEASONAL AFFECTIVE DISORDER (SAD)
HOMEOPATHIC REMEDY

Sol (Imponderables)

There is a homeopathic remedy, Sol, which is actually made from potentiated sunlight. Sol belongs to a group of remedies made from energies such as x-rays and spectrum colors, individually and in combinations. Because of their subtle composition, extreme even for a homeopath, these peculiar remedies, known as the Imponderables,[5] produce allopathic as well as homeopathic effects. Sol may be useful in dealing with disorientation resulting from both an excess of sunlight, as in a heatstroke, and with a deficiency, as in "sundowning" behavior, discussed later in this chapter in the section on Alzheimer's disease.

SMELL DIMENSION ILLNESS: DEPRESSION

The prolonged disaffection of chronically depressed individuals signals their disorientation in time and their loss of connection to the source of breath. Sighing (a junior version of wheezing), commonly found among depressed individuals, expresses a desire to exhale away painful past experiences. Yawning (a junior version of serial gasping) pertains to boredom and anxiety with the current state of affairs. The overinhalation action of yawning may be a subconsciously practiced act intended to propel us away from the present moment into the future.

SMELL DIMENSION ILLNESS: DEPRESSION
HOMEOPATHIC REMEDY

Natrium muriaticum

Let us consider a female patient for whom the homeopathic remedy Natrum muriaticum (sodium chloride, or table salt) is beneficial. As a girl she would have been described as possessing an emotionally sensitive nature. For our purposes, this indicates enjoyment of poetry, a tendency to form powerful emotional attachments, a readiness to cry or laugh easily, and a capacity to be profoundly moved by significant events. At the age of twelve, this girl suffers the loss of her mother with whom she had enjoyed an especially strong bond.

The grief she subsequently undergoes proves difficult to process. Well into adulthood she is marked by a diminished ability to cry openly, accept consolation, or display emotion outwardly. She has allergies, perfectionist tendencies, a habit of smiling inappropriately when relating sad events, and insomnia resulting from distressing memories.

Unlike psychologists, homeopaths are not restricted to noting only mental and emotional symptoms; specific physical symptoms can be included as well. Thus, a headache or eye pain made worse from exposure to the sun, back pain ameliorated by strong pressure, a tendency to constipation or hemorrhoids, and cravings for salt and chocolate, are included in our subject's profile.

For our patient, pushing through the intensely experienced feeling of abandonment after the death of her mother is a nonviable option; doing so is perceived as an act of disloyalty to her mother. Compounding the patient's difficulty in allowing grieving to progress is a second dilemma: If her crying could ever adequately express the depth of her grief, her tears would never end. In her suppressed state as a grown woman she retains a susceptibility to overriding sadness and melancholy. All that is needed for an episode of depression to be triggered is for the pertinent hot button to be pushed, which almost any experience suggestive of loss accomplishes. Our subject's emotional life is a radical disjunct summed up by the statement: "I am desperate for intimacy, but keep it at arm's length."

Many caregivers would justifiably determine that our patient is clinically depressed. Homeopathic and dimensional reasoning, however, lends further perspective to this diagnosis. To need Natrum muriaticum, meaning to be under the influence of sodium chloride, denotes a state of self-containedness, a concept familiar in regard to the relationship between excess salt intake and hypertension. Salt holds water in the cells, thereby increasing arterial pressure. Our Natrum muriaticum patient may be compared to a besieged country that expends excessive resources defending its periphery. Although the country appears strong outwardly, it is tender and weak within its borders.

Perhaps a means other than Natrum muriaticum can help to further resolve our patient's delusional need to misappropriate resources and overprotect her interior. With successful treatment, our patient breaks through her overattachment to the past. She begins to experience the fullness of the present moment, and recaptures her orientation in time.

SMELL DIMENSION ILLNESS: ALZHEIMER'S DISEASE "A BROKEN COMPASS"

Alzheimer's disease has been defined as an irreversible, progressive, debilitating brain disorder resulting in the death of brain cells, dementia, and, eventually, the death of the individual. In the year 2000, it was estimated to affect between three and four million Americans, and it was already the third most costly disease in the U.S. Senescence is the greatest risk factor. With 78 million baby boomers beginning to turn 60 years of age, in the year 2007, a new case of Alzheimer's disease developed approximately every 72 seconds. If the trend continues, by mid-century this will occur every 33 seconds.[6]

Alzheimer's disease destroys our bearings by spiraling like a tornado upwards through the brain. Although the reasoning functions located in the cerebrum succumb in time, the hippocampus and orientation are the first to be attacked. Early research on autopsied brains of individuals suffering damage to the hippocampus reveal the crucial importance of this region of the limbic system to the maintenance of orientation, or frame of reference.[7] If the Alzheimer's patient startles or becomes terrified when he hears a telephone ring, it is because he no longer associates the ringing sound with a telephone. If a fire starts in his apartment, he may be unable to link the presence of flames with danger. As disorientation advances, the meaning of familiar words drops away from their sounds.

Recent research suggests that hippocampal spatial firing patterns and neuronal responses to task-relevant stimuli are highly sensitive to context; furthermore, spatial memories derived from experiences that occurred in familiar surroundings before the illness set in may possibly be independent of the hippocampus.[8,9]

A study, begun in 1991, by the National Institute on Aging, enrolled 678 members of sisters of a religious congregation (called the "Nun Study"); the study followed the cohort of sisters for several years in order to research early-, mid-, and late-life risk factors for brain diseases. Results of the study suggested that the risk factors for Alzheimer's disease, such as its main genetic marker, the apolipoprotein E isoform ApoE4, age, and linguistic ability, are strongly associated with memory impairment, but do not convert memory impairment into full-blown Alzheimer's disease. The researchers inferred from this that major risk factors occur very early in the cascade of events leading to Alzheimer's and that there is a critical time, before the symptoms appear, when interventions can have the greatest effect on preventing brain diseases.[10]

Until 2010, there were no clear-cut tests to diagnose Alzheimer's illness during life, although the presence of the risk factor ApoE4, while it did not prove that a dementia is associated with Alzheimer's, might supplementally indicate the likelihood that it is. In 2010, a team of researchers, using the U.S. Alzheimer's Disease Neuroimaging Initiative database, reported that three biomarkers derived from cerebrospinal fluid correctly classified 90 percent of patients diagnosed with Alzheimer's disease, and were also found in more than one-third of cognitively normal adults; they concluded that these protein biomarkers "are true indicators of the pathogenic process at an early stage."[11]

Two independent research studies in mice, carried out at Columbia and Harvard universities, found that Alzheimer's disease starts in the entorhinal cortex of the brain, where dying cells are filled with an abnormal, "distorted" protein known as tau; the tau then spreads the disease, like an infection, moving in an anatomically-defined pattern along networks connecting vulnerable neurons.[12]

Although an understanding of the genomics of Alzheimer's disease is just beginning, it is becoming clear that Alzheimer's is an independent, complex clinical entity associated with multiple genetic defects, arising either by mutations or by susceptibility to environmental factors.[13]

Inherited genes and chromosomal mutations are found to be correlated in particular with late-onset Alzheimer's disease. As will be argued in the chapter on the dimension of hearing, inherited susceptibilities to illness represent the memory of encounters with pathology having consolidated within Kidney Yang. One recent study comparing the dietary evolution of chimpanzees with humans suggested that in humans, ApoE has evolved over millions of years as an evolutionary adaptation to meat-eating, humans originally having been plant eaters. Further, the ApoE4 allele is considered ancestral within humans, and exists in all human populations within the range of less than 1% to 45%. The ApoE4 variant hastens degenerative changes in the arteries and brain and, depending on the population, can present a greater than ten-fold excess risk of Alzheimer's disease.[14] Although a meat-rich diet proffers the advantages of greater concentrations of calories and micronutrients, the paradox of this diet, according to the study's author, is that "The greater meat consumption of longer-lived humans" with its correspond-ing "greater fat and caloric intake is associated with accelerated pathogenesis and shortened lifespan." Moreover, although the largely plant-eating chimpanzees studied in captivity rarely live longer than 50 years, they "present a lower inci-dence of cancer, ischemic heart disease, and neurodegeneration than current hu-man populations."[14]

To stretch the paradox even further, in 2010, Yian Gu and colleagues at Co-lumbia University published a four-year cohort study of 2,148 patients, ages 65 years and older, that identified a protective dietary pattern associated with a 40% lower risk of developing Alzheimer's. This diet was rich in olive oil, nuts, fish, poultry, fruits, dark and green leafy and cruciferous vegetables, and avoided high-fat dairy products, red meat, and organ meat; in other words, a dietary pattern high in omega-3 and omega-6 fatty acids, vitamins E and B-12, and folate.[15]

A 2010 report from a team of Italian researchers compared the gut microbes in healthy children from Florence, Italy, and from a rural African village in Burki-na Faso, where the children still ate foods similar to those eaten 10,000 years ago, at the time of the birth of agriculture—that is, a diet high in fiber, cereals, legumes, vegetables, and nonanimal protein. The researchers found that com-pared to the Italian children, who ate foods typical of a Western diet—high in animal protein, fat, and sugar, and low in fiber—the Burkina Faso children had more populous and diverse gut microflora that protected them from allergies and diseases such as Crohn's disease, inflammatory bowel disorder, and diarrhea. The study results suggested that "diet has a dominant role over other possible variables such as ethnicity, sanitation, hygiene, geography, and climate, in shaping gut mi-crobiota." The researchers further hypothesized that the "consumption of sugar, animal fat, and calorie-dense foods in industrialized countries is rapidly limiting the adaptive potential of the microbiota."[16]

Clinical study also indicates that Alzheimer's disease embodies the dimension of smell's central liability, disorientation. Indeed, individuals who progress toward Alzheimer's dementia undergo a distortion and loss of the sense of smell (which they themselves may fail to register), perhaps already in the early stages of the illness.[17]

The dimension of smell, as the ancient Taoists noted, is associated with a specific flavor, "umami."[18] The taste of umami ranges from pungent to acrid. Detection of umami by means of smell and taste indicates the presence of amino acids, such as those contained in broiled meats and monosodium glutamate. TCM reasoning indicates that sensitivity to, or desire for, this flavor is medically significant.

Moderate consumption of umami-flavored foods or exposure to pungent aromas strengthens the dimension of smell and enhances orientation; but excessive consumption of umami-flavored foods undermines orientation. An intense craving for meat may predispose us to, or result from, excessive meat consumption; in either case, a high demand for umami reflects an energetic disharmony.

SMELL DIMENSION ILLNESS: ALZHEIMER'S DISEASE
HOMEOPATHIC REMEDIES

Sol (Imponderables)

The literal meaning of orientation is to face eastward, toward the Orient, in the direction from which the sun rises. At sundown, when Alzheimer's patients are most disoriented, they exhibit a tendency to wander that is so commonplace, skilled nursing home staff refer to it as "sundowning." In every respect, sundowning is the reverse of orientation. Sol, a homeopathic remedy made from sunlight, introduced earlier in the discussion of SAD, may prove to be of use with regard to sundowning and related behaviors. Sol's remedy picture includes features very specific to Alzheimer's patients: easily frightened, fatigued toward the end of the day, indecisive, restless, irritable, and, of course, disorientated.

Alumina

Homeopathic materia medica helps us to understand Alzheimer's disease by modeling the disease as a failure to resolve core issues. An Alumina remedy state results from either exposure or response to life events. In the case of exposure, the remedy picture reflects aluminum's chemical toxicity and the effect on the brain's neurotransmitters; as a response, the remedy indicates that a susceptibility to the Alumina mind-set has been promoted. Individuals in need of Alumina manifest a powerful confusion, a feeling akin to having two heads. This is induced by events having led them to compromise their will and suffer loss of independence.

The evolution of an Alumina mind-set can also invite neuropathology. An elderly woman suffering from multiple sclerosis was in my care as a patient. As a young woman, she had been pushed into marrying a man she did not care for by an alliance of the man himself with her older sister. Use of the remedy Alumina resulted in a greater willingness on her part to hold a conversation, in mitigating her sense of confusion, in a slight, but definite, improvement in her coordination, and in a generally more relaxed demeanor.

SMELL DIMENSION ILLNESS: BRAIN-WASTING PRION DISEASES

Prions, or "proteinaceous infectious particles," are peculiar and unique disease-causing proteins, found by the neurologist Stanley B. Prusiner, in the early 1980s; Prusiner called the protein PrP, for "prion protein." For reasons and by means as yet unknown, prions are able to invert their structure, replicate, and change their shape, converting normal protein molecules into dangerous ones. The known prion diseases, all fatal, are also called spongiform encephalopathies because the proliferation of prions leaves gaping holes in the brain tissue of mammals. The most common form, found in sheep and goats, is called scrapie, a term arising from the animals' need to scrape off their wool or hair because of an intense symptomatic itch. Bovine spongiform encephalopathy, named Mad Cow disease, was identified in cows in Great Britain in 1986; the source of the disease was found to be a food supplement fed to the cows made from ground-up carcasses of cattle and sheep, which may have been infected with a brain-wasting disease.

In humans, prion diseases are infectious, neurodegenerative diseases that have a uniquely wide range of phenotypes and can be sporadic, familial or inherited, or acquired by infection. In fact, the great variability of phenotypes has made it difficult to identify prion diseases.[19] Some prion diseases, like kuru, are found only in highlanders living in Papua New Guinea; it has been assumed that they acquired kuru through ritual cannibalism. Since the practice has stopped, kuru has virtually disappeared. Other prion diseases, like Creutzfeldt-Jakob disease (CJD), occur worldwide, usually sporadically. About 10% of CJD is known to be inherited; the rest is iatrogenically transmitted, in some cases by eating contaminated meat. Scrapie, CJD, and kuru have all been shown to be transmissible and fatal.[20]

By 2007, over 200 cases of a virulent CJD departure, variant Creutzfeldt-Jakob disease (vCJD), had been reported in humans, primarily in the United Kingdom. The clear evidence showed that vCJD was transmitted to humans by eating prion-contaminated beef.[21] Yet more virulent strains of fatal prion diseases in humans, such as the new variant Creutzfeldt-Jakob (nvCJD), are being found.[22]

According to Prusiner, in 1995,

> We do know with certainty that cleavage of scrapie PrP is what produces PrP fragments that accumulate as plaques in the brains of some patients. Those aggregates resemble plaques seen in Alzheimer's disease, although the Alzheimer's clumps consist of a different protein. The PrP plaques are a useful sign of prion infection, but they seem not to be a major cause of impairment. In many people and animals with prion disease, the plaques do not arise at all.[20]

Prusiner's observation regarding PrP's relationship to plaques was investigated a step further in research by Laurén and associates, published in February 2009.[23] According to these researchers, prion proteins appear to interact with amyloid-beta from early-stage plaques. In this study, however, they found no evidence that the prion proteins actually fold into an abnormal shape or cause Alzheimer's.

Following along this line of work, a study by Ghoshal and colleagues at Washington University School of Medicine, published in October 2009, reported for the first time that three persons from a family in Illinois who had died from an inherited form of CJD, had the same type of amyloid plaques as those found in the identical brain regions of Alzheimer's patients. According to the researchers, "The finding adds to other, earlier evidence suggesting that the misfolded protein believed to cause CJD, known as a prion, appears to play a role in the Alzheimer's disease process."[24]

Apparently, Jews of Libyan descent have an incidence of familial CJD (fCJD) which is about 100 times higher than that of the general population. Initially attributed to consumption of the brains of sheep, the suggested origins of the fCJD identified in this population have included a mutation on the prion protein gene as well as abnormal stress and anxiety levels among the healthy fCJD mutation carriers.[25,26]

SMELL DIMENSION ILLNESS:
CANCER OF THE BREAST AND LARGE INTESTINE:
FRAMESHIFT MUTATIONS

When we characterize a particular trait or disease as genetic, we generally mean that its emergence is "preordained." Expressing a biochemical disorder, or glitch, the genetic trait or disease lies outside our ordinary sphere of influence. What so frightens people about cancer is its consequent uncontrollability. Some mechanism goes haywire in the program according to which cells normally divide and cease dividing. Previously typical cells begin to multiply rapidly and invasively in a process that nerve and hormonal action are at a loss to control.

But not all the news is bleak. It is now clear that an important distinction exists between our genetic design, or genotype, and healthful or unhealthful gene expression, or phenotype.[27] The phenotype may be modified by lifestyle as well as by activation of the mind-body connection.

We find that centeredness combats disorientation, even at the genetic level. Both the colon and the breast are vulnerable to orientation-related issues because they are components of the large intestines and chest, anatomic regions associated with the dimension of smell, and noted for the unusual degree of chaos governing cell replication within its attendant malignancies. Forms of these cancers result from a particularly devastating type of mutation known as a frameshift, representing disorientation occurring at the genetic level.

Frameshift Mutations

When disorientation manifests at the linguistic level, the sounds of words cease to express their proper meanings; like a worn-out fabric, the context of our mental associations has fallen apart. Genetic replication can be likened to a linguistic process that requires a context of meaning to be sustained.

A nucleotide equals a frame that is being read. In terms of a linguistic analogy, the frame equals the context of meaning. During gene replication, messenger RNA, using the DNA as a template, copies a series of instructions for protein synthesis. The expression of these instructions is virtually a prose sentence in which codons (a specific sequence of three DNA bases within a gene, responsible for directing the synthesis of amino acid molecules possessing highly specific molecular structures that are vital for the formation of proteins) function as the constituent words. The nucleotides themselves may be thought of as syllables.

In a related, though far less dangerous, mutation than a frameshift mutation, the single nucleotide polymorphism, substitution of an incorrect nucleotide during transcription of DNA bases in the production of messenger RNA, generally alters only a single triplet group, leaving the remaining sequence of codons unaltered. This is the equivalent of writing a set of instructions for the manufacture of a defective shoe, which, when it leaves the assembly line, is found to lack a specific feature such as eye holes.

In the much more serious mutation known as a frameshift, which involves the bases in an entire sequence of codons within a molecule of messenger RNA following the deletion (or addition) of a single nucleotide, the frame shifts (forward or backward), leaving the following sequence of bases scrambled. A frameshift produces the equivalent of a set of shoe-manufacture instructions that somewhere in the middle of the paragraph degenerates into total nonsense. When the instructions are followed to the letter, an object unrecognizable as a shoe rolls off the assembly line.

A frameshift is thus a mutagenic change that brings an unusual degree of disorganization to the gene packet involved in genetic replication. It leaves nothing but chaos in its wake. Frameshift mutations, which almost always result in the synthesis of an abnormal protein, produce dysfunction ranging from mild abnormality to malignancy.

Acridine, a hydrocarbon compound, a by-product of coal combustion used in the manufacture of dyes, biological stains, and antibacterial agents, is a mutagen and the most acrid gas known. Positively-charged acridine dyes bind directly to the DNA; they sandwich themselves between stacked base pairs of DNA, inserting or deleting one base pair in DNA, resulting in frameshift mutations.

The Wellcome Trust Sanger Institute's Cancer Genome Project currently lists over 75 cancer genes, involving the entire range of tumor types and cancer syndromes, that are characterized by frameshift mutations.[28]

A BROADER PERSPECTIVE

Although few among us, if any, are sufficiently advanced that we can command perfect orientation at the biochemical level, we can limit the risk of predisposal to a genetic disorientation through healthy living.

Pressing as genetic and biochemical questions are, they reflect an overly narrow perspective. The virus we seek may long remain shadowy; the prion, mysterious; the toxin or mutant gene ultimately responsible for turning our healthy brains into sponge, continually beyond reach. Preservation of our mental health requires a shift to a broader and more compassionate perspective. A resolution to respect animals, and to follow the diet nature has given us to eat is in order. Within our capacity to perform, a simple adjustment can deliver a valuable benefit: the reinstatement and preservation of our bearings.

The compassionate perspective is well described by what the Taoists call the Po, a kind of universal soul encompassing all things that breathe. We visit the Po when we access the dimension of smell by practicing awareness of our breathing. Our most precious commodity, the air, is shared by all, and in equal measure. Visits to Po consciousness teach us to have regard for others. In doing so, we learn that no success, failure, profit, loss, survival, or death is ever completely an individual matter, and that universal brotherhood is more than a slogan.

THE SMELL DIMENSION: PERSONAL THERAPEUTIC PRACTICES AND MASTERS OF EXPRESSION

Various therapeutic practices can help promote health within the sense dimension of smell. **Table 1** on the following page shows several of these practices.

Masters throughout history have strongly expressed either the positive or negative poles of the sense dimension of smell. **Table 2** lists a few who exemplified one or the other side of the centeredness-disorientation axis, the core issue of the dimension of smell.

Table 1. Smell Dimension: Health-promoting Practices

Develop a strategic capability	Meditate; harmonize the breath
Minimize scent pollution	Process grief, then move on
Preserve clean air	Practice martial arts
Nurture the mother of smell, *Taste*: "Identify and accept genuine challenges"	Nurture family ties

Table 2. Examples of Masters of the Sense Dimension of Smell

NEGATIVE POLE: DISORIENTATION	POSITIVE POLE: CENTEREDNESS
Pablo Picasso: fractured space in Cubist paintings	Meditation instructors: "Being in the here and now"
Stan Brakhage: fractured time in experimental films	Zen Master Suzuki Roshi (*Zen Mind, Beginner's Mind*)
Alain Resnais: (*Last Year at Marienbad*)	Martial arts masters from Tai Qi families: centered awareness of danger, direction, and possibility
	Morehei Uyeshiba, founder of Aikido

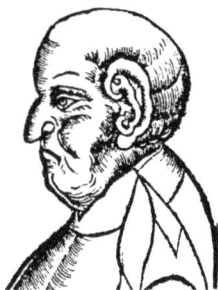

CHAPTER SIX

THE DIMENSION OF HEARING

THE SENSE DIMENSION OF HEARING

PHASE	WATER
ORGAN	KIDNEYS
CORE ISSUE	CONSOLIDATION–ENTROPY

Hearing is the ability to interpret audible sound, based on the collection and transformation of fluctuations in pressure. The cognitive aspect of hearing—the selective act of listening—has no equivalent among the other four senses. Within the cacophony of surrounding sound, we pay attention to what interests us and turn a deaf ear to all else. To an extent greater than with any other sense, hearing requires that we discriminate between what we permit to pass through and what we do not. This ability to shift attention within sound may result from a distinct neurological feature: As opposed to other sensory pathways, the auditory pathway is bilateral. Sensory fibers issuing from each of the two auditory cochlea within the inner ear are both crossed and uncrossed. Each cochlea is represented in both hemispheres of the brain. Even if we were deaf in one ear our hearing would remain stereophonic.

Our inner-ear mechanism is an arrangement of intricate tubing filled with fluid. It has many similarities with a system of hair and canals found in fish; arch-like tissues found in the middle ear resemble gill-like slits. The human middle ear appears to have evolved from the first two arches (and the neck structure containing them). This system, known as the lateral-line canal, allows fish while swimming to detect variations in water pressure and the presence of moving objects such as predators. Our modern hearing sense is consequently an elaboration on the kinesthetic awareness of fish moving about in water. In order to make the transmission of sound more efficient, the external auditory canal connecting the outer ear to the eardrum is lined by a combination of epithelial and periosteum tissue. A pervasive theme of water involves an energetic interplay within our body between epithelial and osseous (bone or periosteum) tissue.

Appropriately, water is profound—in TCM, a deep Phase. Water's domain is like a sex-and-death drama celebrated by philosophers, the originators of the Greek myths, the tragic playwrights Sophocles, Euripedes, O'Neill, Ibsen, and scientists of the mind such as Sigmund Freud and Sándor Ferenczi (postulator of a conflict between Eros, the life instinct and Thanatos, the death instinct).

Hearing allows simultaneous production and perception of sense data, meaning that we can hear self-produced sounds. The vibration of our own voice lends resonance to our thoughts and emotions; for example, meditation states entered into by chanting are vibrant.

Hearing also arranges sound qualities associated with each of the senses. The quality specifically connected with hearing is pitch; the level of pitch denotes the frequency of a sound vibration. In Eastern religion a specific pitch also activates a chakra, one of seven, vertically-arrayed, mind-body energy centers within the body. In TCM, a vibration produced and directed towards the dantien center, the body's center of gravity and storage center for Qi, located just below and behind the navel, can generate desirable, energy-integrating, and spiritually-grounding effects.

Perhaps life began as the Bible says: "In the beginning was the Word." If so, then the universe was created because of Logos, a primordial vocalization imbued with meaning. If the Word preceded all else, who or what was there to hear and attend to it? If nothing, then the primordial Word must have contained the seeds of its own response: a capability to separate, differentiate, consolidate, and perpetuate whatever is its own.

We hear a calling, a commitment. In spiritual terms, the health of the hearing dimension requires us to attend to what might be called the voice of God, a directive that the life mission which was uniquely consolidated within each of us is carried out. In physical terms, this mission may be the expression of a pattern transmitted from one or more ancestors that has consolidated within our lineage. Bert Hellinger, psychoanalyst, former Catholic priest, and cofounder of Constellation therapy, with its roots in existential phenomenology, Zulu ancestral spirit culture, and family therapy, postulated that betrayal of the ancestral presence, or the actual but denied ostracism of a deceased relative, exacts injury to our health.[1]

THE KIDNEYS IN TRADITIONAL CHINESE MEDICINE

Although they lacked a tradition of rational philosophy, the ancient Chinese did develop philosophically grounded, conceptual tools with which to diagnose and treat illness. The Chinese modeling of the Kidney function, for example, reflects a rational framework for how, within living things, biological information is organized and perpetuated. Accordingly, cell development and replication, the immune response, hypersensitivity, genetic predisposition, and also evolution are found to emanate from the core Kidney consolidation function.

The Kidney is conceived of in TCM as the root of life, providing the foundation for Yin (Water) and Yang (Fire). It also governs the balance between these polar-opposite Phases. As the ruler of Water, the Kidneys oversee the distribution and circulation of nutritive fluids and the excretion of impure fluids. Yet the Kidneys also supply an accessory, Fire, known variously as Ming Men Fire, Source Qi, or Kidney Yang. This Fire aids in digestion, fluid transport, warming of the body, and retention of urine by the bladder. The Yang force of the Kidneys is also charged with holding down or providing a root for Qi derived from air inhaled by the lungs. Failure of this function leads to shortness of breath and coughing.

The Kidneys are the storehouse of Essence (Jing), which rules the bones, controls reproductive functions, and controls the overall life cycle of development and decline. Bone, marrow, teeth, and brain tissue are all considered to be influenced by Jing, as are conception and pregnancy. Excessive sexual activity and too many or too closely spaced pregnancies deplete Jing. From a biomedical perspective, Jing's life-cycle control would be attributed to our genetic material. In TCM, prenatal Jing is inherited from the parents, and it is supplemented with postnatal Jing derived from food.

The Kidneys and their paired organ, the Urinary Bladder, belong to the Phase of Water. The Water Phase is associated with the ears and hearing, and with the emotion of fear and the vocal sound of groaning.

The signs and symptoms of Kidney disorders in TCM include a weak constitution, birth defects, bone pathologies, malformed teeth, retarded mental development, poor memory, deafness, abnormal sexual drive, infertility, menstrual problems, coldness, pain in the low back and knees, urinary dysfunctions, edema, shortness of breath, asthma, and chronic diarrhea.

HEARING DIMENSION CORE ISSUE: THE CONSOLIDATION–ENTROPY AXIS

Kidney Essence, Reproduction, and the Interplay Between Yin and Yang

In TCM theory, the ears are the opening of the Kidneys, which control reproduction. The ancient Chinese are not the only ones to hold that the ears possess a relationship to reproduction. In early Christian theology, the Archangel Gabriel's announcement to Mary of her pregnancy generated speculation that the breath of the Holy Ghost entered her through her ear, a notion that Ernest Jones undertook to investigate psychoanalytically.[2] Greek mythology relates that the goddess Athena was birthed through the ear of Zeus.

Let us explore this relationship further within TCM theory, in which the primeval energies of Yin and Yang can be expressed in terms of souls. The Yang soul is the Hun, or Ethereal Soul; it is nonmaterial and immortal. The Hun manifests our individual will and sense of purpose. Its Yin counterpart is the Po, or Corporeal Soul. The Po relates to the material aspect of our existence and is mortal, passing into nonexistence with the demise of our body.

During fertilization, or conception, Yang from the universe projects the Hun into the receptive egg, or Po. The two united souls form a living being whose life energy is fueled by an unbroken connection with Yang streaming forth from its source in the universe.

In the course of fetal development, the Po is said to take up residence in the Lungs. At the time of birth, the Po oversees the young organism's activation of its lungs; its orientation to material energy sources, such as air, light, and food; its coordination with the various functions of its organs. The Hun inhabits the Liver from where it provides motivation and spiritual direction.

Connected to the universal source of life energy, Yang is maintained in a space between the two Kidneys known as the Gate of Life. Yang may be thought of as voltage, a power to infuse organic tissue with life energy.

That Yang is infinite and Yin is limited is indicated physically by the fact that healthy males can produce viable sperm indefinitely, while females possess a limited amount of eggs. In accordance with the principle of Logos, infinitely surging Yang energy must eventually be articulated and create and detach from itself a Yin counterpart, Kidney Essence, which in its active form is called Jing, and which takes up residence in the left Kidney.

The remaining Yang portion, known as Kidney Fire, takes up residence in the right Kidney, from where it can fulfill its mission of infusing energy and generating the sexual drive in the new organism.

The finite Jing, unstinting in its efforts to separate, differentiate, consolidate, and perpetuate its position within the new young organism, is haunted by the primal anxiety of loss of substantiality by entropy and a return to the emptiness of the great Tao.

Kidney Fire's anxiety pertains to its responsibility to guard reproductive energy in its material form: the Yang must be kept firm so that erections are not lost; the sperm must be consolidated so that it does not dribble away during the night or through premature ejaculation. If the Kidneys are functionally weak or the new organism becomes frightened, the Kidney Fire's inability to help with breathing also causes it anxiety, for the Kidneys must grasp the Qi of inhaled air, pulling it downward into the lungs.

Kidney Fire also provides heat for the organism's breakdown of foodstuffs and metabolism. As if in response, a portion of the acquired Essence of life—the by-products of metabolism—is stored within the body where it can supplement the limited supply of congenital Kidney Essence and be available for emergency use by all the organs of the body.

Health within the dimension of hearing thus demands that we reconcile the universe's two great forces: on the one hand, entropy (the dissolution of structure; death); on the other, consolidation (the gathering, organizing, and self-perpetuation of knowledge, the machinery of procreation). In somatic terms, health within hearing requires that our energy be integrated, efficient, and genetically viable.

CONSOLIDATION

The ancient Chinese texts state that the Kidney rules the water channels and the bones. From a sense-dimensional standpoint, the water channels and the bones are one and the same. However, both epithelial tissue—which includes the exocrine glands (sweat, salivary and other)—and bone (osseous) tissue—including the periosteum or bone covering and the teeth—provide separation. Given the body's need to establish boundaries between different tissues, the epithelium and bone tissues express opposing receptive and repellent borders. Both types of tissues, however, are the responsibility of Jing.

The epithelium is a moist, semipermeable tissue, a membrane designed for biochemical transport or optimal communication between neighboring tissues. The epithelium pertains to the water channels, in which case it is known as Kidney Yin, an energy function that describes the health of the exocrine glands, the adrenal glands, the bladder, and the kidneys themselves. Osseous tissue pertains to the bone or periosteum and allows little interaction with neighboring tissue. Osseous tissue represents structure, support, and protection.

The skeletal frame maintains our stability in its Yang aspect, meaning structurally. Further, the vestibular nervous system, whose principal components are found within the inner ear, maintains our stability in its Yin aspect. The derangement of this system is known as Menière's syndrome.

In TCM, Jing undertakes responsibility, under the ancient textual name of Yuan (or source) Qi, for the so-called extraordinary organs in the body. These extraordinary organs are the bone marrow, the uterus, the spinal cord, the blood vessels, the gall bladder, and the brain. Via Yuan Qi the Kidneys are directly involved with reproductive and menstrual functions, production of circulatory and menstrual blood, spinal integrity, bone density, and brain function. Jing's involvement in reproduction is strong, because in a fertilized egg the opposing natures of epithelial and osseous tissues are temporarily reconciled (as bone and membrane at this stage are indistinguishable). During reproduction, Jing—if only for a single generation—can resist the feared entropy.

ENTROPY

The ancient Chinese conceived of the process of maturation and aging chiefly as the depletion and loss of Jing. Jing is minimally stressed when Yin and

Yang (fluid and energy) are abundant and well-managed: epithelial tissue then remains soft and moist, while bone tissue stays hard and dry. Ongoing stress, however, may create profound imbalances in these tissues, for example, severe diarrhea in epithelial membrane and osteoporosis in bone tissue. The biochemical community increasingly recognizes that stress is a contributing factor in human disease, especially depression, cardiovascular disease, and HIV/AIDS.[3]

Normal aging can also occur through increased susceptibility to pathogenic cold, injuring the physical body, the container of Yang. With the weakening of the capability to manage the body, the power of Yang is also diminished in the body; the sexual drive is reduced and other symptoms may appear: pallor, cold limbs, soreness and weakness of the lower back and knees, night-time urination, tinnitus, vertigo, and a white-coated tongue. The homeopathic remedy exemplifying this aging process is Selenium.

HEARING DIMENSION: CHRONIC ILLNESSES

HEARING DIMENSION ILLNESS: ADDICTION

According to the National Institute on Drug Abuse (NIDA) of the National Institutes of Health, "Addiction is defined as a chronic, relapsing brain disease that is characterized by compulsive drug seeking and use, despite harmful consequences. It is considered a brain disease because drugs change the brain—they change its structure and how it works. These brain changes can be long lasting. . . ."[4] NIDA further states that although the initial use of drugs is voluntary and highly pleasurable, over time the feelings of pleasure become less pleasurable, and the drug user is compelled to take higher or more frequent doses of the drug in order to feel "normal." Scientists believe that because drug-addiction changes the way the brain works in areas of judgment, decision-making, learning, memory, and behavior control, the drug abuser is eventually compelled to act compulsively and destructively. NIDA estimates that genetic factors, including mental disorders and the effects of the environment on gene expression and function, account for some 40% to 60% of the vulnerability to addiction; environmental factors, such as a dysfunctional home life, intemperate parents, abuse, peer pressure, poor social skills, and academic failure, account for the rest:[4] in other words, nature and nurture.

HEARING DIMENSION ILLNESS: ADDICTION
HOMEOPATHIC REMEDIES

Do our insights into the dimension of hearing in this chapter have implications for the treatment of addiction? In alcohol addiction, for example, a person discovers that drinking provides an escape from psychic pain. His subsequent attempts at self-control in order to eliminate the negative effects of drinking become a psychic pain in and of themselves, prompting further drinking. This self-reinforcing dynamic spirals in intensity until it finally glyphs onto the Kidney Yang, where its consolidation within the dimension of hearing promotes or reflects self-referential patterns of thought.

Mercurius, Syphilinum, Lanthanides

Syphilitic remedies, such as Mercurius (quicksilver) and the nosode Syphilinum, are often used by homeopaths in the treatment of alcoholism. In addition, a larger class of remedies, the Lanthanides, resonates with the consolidation and self-referential nature of the dimension of hearing. The Dutch homeopath, Jan Scholten, in his 2005 book, *Secret Lanthanides*, explored the Lanthanides, a group of elements found at the lower end of the periodic table of elements, for their use as homeopathic remedies.[5] The still controversial Lanthanides are described in detail in Chapter 3 on touch, in the aurum series' section on homeopathic remedies for hypertension. Individuals in need of these remedies and their salts are recognizable by the following qualities: inwardness, a proclivity for self-referential thinking, a likelihood of possessing a singular secret, a tendency to be a searcher—in particular, issues concerning autonomy and addiction.[6]

Lachesis mutatis

Lachesis mutatis (venom of the bushmaster snake) is a remedy that homeopaths often use to help patients who are susceptible to alcohol. Lachesis individuals are intense and passionate, yet also suppressed. As the throat represents a critical boundary in the body between the head, the repository of mentally-directed suppression, and the trunk, the repository of physical needs, Lachesis people are prone to having sensations of choking and strangulation that may develop into asthmatic breathing. They also can endure numerous chest and heart symptoms, particularly palpitations, and they can feel quite hot. Their skin is sensitive and can also bruise easily. Emotionally, they fear snakes, are anxious, tend to be jealous, and are prone to suspicion and premonitions. Because Lachesis mutatis is made from the dilution of deadly snake venom, their anxiety relates on a profound level to the fear of death.

Lachesis mutatis expresses a dilemma that Sigmund Freud in his book, *Civilization and Its Discontents*, identifies as the central problem of modern civilization. Freud asks: How can we reconcile the two great opposing forces in human nature, that is, the primitive, instinctual desire to procreate, and civilization's demand that we repress the expression of our physical need? The Lachesis state resolves Freud's posited dilemma, albeit dysfunctionally and destructively, either by illness or by alcoholism. My own practice shows, however, that rather than being the core enigma of human nature, "the expression of instinct versus the suppression of instinct" and its associated reprieve in alcoholism, presents only one of many human dilemmas possessing the potential to crystallize and consolidate within our lineage.

TCM and Lachesis mutatis

In TCM, an analysis of the Phases indicates that the Lachesis state reflects an excess of Fire energy (heart palpitations, passion, feeling of heat) conjoined with a deficiency of Water (anxiety, premonitions, suppression of sexuality). In this instance, Fire compensates for Water: As drinking alcohol escalates, the pathological cycle intensifies; the alcohol drives water out of the cells, further depleting the Kidney's ability to control the Heart's spirit and blood.

Addictions, especially to alcohol, are usually refractory to cure. In my experience, addiction represents an ongoing spiritual challenge. For those who have an inherited susceptibility to alcohol, acceptance of spiritual values and a spiritual purpose enhances the body's Yang and helps conserve the Kidney's Essence. This acceptance of spiritual values, however, helps to subdue, but not entirely eliminate, the hard-wired desperation that fuels alcoholism.

In addition to the remedies described here, numerous others merit use or study in relation to the various aspects of addiction. Prominent among these are Aurum metallicum, Nux vomica, Sulphuricum acidum, Medorrhinum, Alcoholus, Cannabis sativa, Apocynum androsaemifolium, and Opium.

HEARING DIMENSION ILLNESS:
LOWER BACK PAIN AND SCOLIOSIS

L ower back pain and acute sprains of the back are common and can sometimes be caused by simple overexertion or stretching of the muscles. Repeated trauma, however, can damage underlying soft tissue, cause herniation of the spinal discs, and even torque the spine.

Lower Back Pain, Scoliosis, and TCM

When a lower-back injury is muscular, TCM describes the trauma as the stagnation of blood and Qi, which may be resolved by the stimulation of Qi and the promotion of blood circulation through acupuncture and homeopathy. A chronic lower-back condition, however, combined with unusual sensitivity to cold, loss of feeling in the lower limbs, and diminished sexual energy, is seen in TCM as a reduction of Kidney Yang. As we have discussed in this chapter, because Yang in the body is dependent on nourishment by Jing or Essence, Kidney Fire is also depleted if Jing is stressed. Therefore, the treatment called for in cases of chronic lower-back pain is the nourishment of Jing and the energizing of Kidney Fire.

In TCM, congenital defects are seen as manifesting a deficiency of Yang, imprinted by stress that has been consolidated and perpetuated within Jing or Essence over the course of generations. Our discussion of Water suggests that Essence is programmed to consolidate and perpetuate what it learns. Thus, a hereditary predisposition to scoliosis, for example, can develop from experiences of traumas undergone by one's ancestors.

Ancestral research in biomedicine is currently emerging in the field of paleovirology, the study of ancient extinct viruses and pathogenic viral infections of human ancestors. Emerman and Malik,[7] of the Fred Hutchinson Cancer Research Center in Seattle, Washington, have largely studied endogenous retroviruses directly identified from their remnants in host genomes. They postulate[7]

> Paleovirology could be viewed as the study of ancient viruses that primate genomes encountered and defeated during the course of evolution. This view emphasizes that our current antiviral repertoire was not optimized to combat present infections, but rather is the product of selection for survival of our species'

past infections. Thus, the selective changes that these antiviral genes incurred during periods of evolutionary pressure might make them less competent to fight modern viral challenges.

Emerman and Malik suggest "that selection to survive the pathogenic effects of these [paleoviruses] has shaped our repertoire of antiviral defenses in ways that impact our resistance or susceptibility to modern-day emerging viruses."[7]

Biomedicine has also coined the term "selfish gene," a gene that has "selfishly" replicated itself, either by acting as a parasite or by cunningly tagging itself as a centromere, in order, like Jing in TCM, to avoid entropy and death. Recent research shows that the most studied of these selfish genes, the 2-μm plasmid, which is ubiquitous in the budding yeast *Saccharomyces cerevisiae*, has survived extinction over millions of years by effectively poaching the centromeric histone Cse4 from its host yeast "to mark its partitioning locus with a centromere tag [revealing] yet another one of the molecular trickeries it performs for achieving chromosome-like fideltity."[8,9]

A Case of Stress Within Water

Located on either side of the spine, the kidneys are an essential part of the urinary system and perform the body's homeostatic functions such as the regulation of electrolytes, the maintenance of the acid-base balance, the regulation of blood pressure, and the filtering of blood. Every day, a person's kidneys process about 200 quarts of blood to sift out about two quarts of waste products and extra water.[10] The kidneys are responsible as well for the reabsorption of water, glucose, and amino acids, and also produce hormones including calcitriol, renin, and erythropoietin.

No wonder the kidneys are key to nourishing and maintaining the health of the body, spine, and lower back, and that any weakening of their ability to function and give sustenance to the body and spine causes the encroachment of entropy, injecting doubt into our ability to stand upright in the world. Kidney weakness amounts to a stressing of the Jing as Yuan Qi, in which Yuan Qi's confidence in nourishing the spine and bones has been undermined.

Emotional issues underlying stress within Water can easily be missed by the practitioner. A patient of mine, coming to see me for an unrelated problem, complained of a recent back strain. "I've been feeling good," she said, "so I did a bit more gardening and housework than I normally do, and I think I pulled a muscle." This, of course, presented a perfectly reasonable account of her back pain. She then mentioned that within a few days she would be visiting her son whose wife had recently given birth to twin boys. The boys had needed minor surgery and were recuperating at home, so there would be a number of family members at the house. My patient related her anxiety at the prospect of being at the center of undue attention as well as being overly relied upon. "I carried that boy first," she mused offhandedly, referring to her son.

I asked her to pause and to repeat what she had said about "carrying that boy first." After giving me a puzzled look, she repeated the words, grew thoughtful, and finally made a mental connection between the expected commotion and the strain of her first pregnancy, with its anticipated repetition in the new grandparent role. My interpretation was that her Yuan Qi had panicked and lost confidence in its ability to nourish the spine. Thus, she had "lost her backbone" and become vulnerable to sprain. The remedy that relieved her spinal distress and helped her to lose her self-consciousness was Silica.

HEARING DIMENSION ILLNESS:
FRACTURES: OVERCALCIFICATION AND BONE LOSS

As stated earlier in this chapter, ascending Kidney Qi grasps the Qi of the air, pulling it downwards into the lungs. The kidneys' investment in the function of the lungs reflects the two organs' shared dependence on the synthesis of one and the same substance, sunshine Vitamin D. As described in the chapter on the dimension of smell, respiration encompasses one's orientation, meaning one's awareness of location and movement, especially in relation to sources of natural light. Plants, being rooted to one spot, are inherently centered. In plants, therefore, movement toward the sun's light (phototropism) and respiration are closely related. Animals and humans, however, are not rooted to a spot on the ground; their vegetative heritage is represented by the bone structure and function, an analog of the plant's central system, and their ability to ambulate obscures the relationship between orientation and respiration.

The evolutionary divergence of plants and animals may be traced back to the creation of separate energy-creating strategies. Within plants, chlorophyll molecules absorb light's energy (photons), and through the functions of various enzymes in the chloroplasts, convert light's energy into chemical energy, which enables the synthesis of carbohydrates out of carbon dioxide (from the air) and water. The chlorophyll protein possesses four porphyrin subunits that are attached to a central metal atom, magnesium. In biochemistry, a metalloprotein is a generic term for a protein that also contains a metal cofactor. The metal may be an isolated ion or may be coordinated with a nonprotein organic compound, such as the porphyrin found in hemoproteins. The presence of heme in every kingdom—bacteria, protists, fungi, plant, and animal—suggests its ancient lineage. The hemoprotein's ability to interact in oxidation-reduction reactions and to transport oxygen is essential for the production of energy in living organisms.

The chloroplast heme requisitions magnesium while the porphoryin heme operating within organisms having a circulatory system requisitions iron, which is centrally located within the hemoglobin protein and without which oxygen cannot be transported from the lungs. Magnesium's key role conjoint with calcium is to consolidate the bones by hardening and rendering them dense (reflecting in TCM the Lungs' investment in the Kidney function). As plants containing chlorophyll are rich in magnesium, this is one good reason to eat our vegetables.

A vestigial connection to phototropism and our vegetative heritage remains with us; this is the synthesis of Vitamin D from exposure to the sun. Although some plants do contain ergocalciferol, a Vitamin D precursor, eating only greens, even those containing calcium, is not a substitute for getting sunshine-activated Vitamin D. Vitamin D is not actually a vitamin but a steroidal enzyme; its deficiency not only undermines bone formation (causing the disease, rickets) but is implicated in developmental dysfunction.

Eating foods with silicon, an essential trace mineral, as well as whole grains, vegetables, legumes, and fruits not only provides sufficient dietary fiber, but also supplies ample calcium and magnesium. Butterfats, because they can bind calcium through a gut saponification process (hydrolization of a fat with alkali to form a soap and glycerol), are to be avoided. Excess consumption of dietary sweets works as a calcium uptake inhibitor, as do carbonated beverages, many of which contain phosphoric or citric acid, harmful ingredients because they act to bind or chelate the calcium, thus reducing its absorption.

HEARING DIMENSION ILLNESS:
FRACTURES: OVERCALCIFICATION AND BONE LOSS
HOMEOPATHIC REMEDIES

Calcarea fluorica

Based on my observations in my practice, I suggest that a specific emotional re-action or stress occurs simultaneously with every physical trauma. If such is the case, which subtle emotional reactions and stresses might underlie the insidious tendency to bone brittleness that so many of us encounter as we age?

The congenital nature of problems encountered within the dimension of hearing tends to override the transformative power of emotional catharsis. Be-cause emotional dynamics within hearing are challenging to detect, we look to the homeopathic database for clues. Calcium fluoride, or fluorspar, is a mineral whose toxicological effect is to produce an excess of bone growth and consequent brittleness. The remedy Calcarea fluorica is beneficial in treating brittleness re-lated to overcalcification.

Calcium fluoride is a white powder, also found in the shape of cubic crystals, that is 51% calcium and 49% fluorine. Homeopathic proving symptoms of Cal-carea fluorica included deficient enamel of the teeth; premature cavities; swelling of the thyroid gland; both hyperthyroidism and hypothyroidism; tardy development of the bones; chronic suppuration of the middle ear; swellings and hard nodes in ligaments (connective tissue), muscles, and tendons; pain in the small of the back; and a variety of skin conditions.[11]

Feldspar, also known as fluorite, along with sulfides of lead, zinc, and some-times silver, is excavated from landscapes where there are high-temperature ther-mal veins. Fluoride thus has an affinity with material acquisition. The psychologi-cal character of calcium fluoride points to a picture of Type A stress that includes indecision and restlessness, but most especially fear of poverty and overemphasis on gaining wealth. The Calcarea fluorica individual's anxiety about money mat-ters, a groundless notion that he will soon fail financially, fits well with the defini-tion of an encounter with entropy: a sense of having lost viability in support of life. On Calcarea fluorica's plus side, its homeopathic provings presented mental quickness and intense concentration, acuteness of the senses, and an unusual feel-ing of personal strength.

In TCM, fluorite tonifies and enhances Yang because the element Fire compensates Water. A the same time, it demonstrates how overvaluing money leads to an eventual depletion of one's Jing or Essence.

Symphytum officinale

Symphytum officinale, from the herbal root comfrey, or knitbone, has been used allopathically as well as homeopathically to help bones to harden and heal, to treat wounds, and to reduce the inflammation associated with sprains and broken bones. Historically, comfrey was also used to treat gastrointestinal illness. However, the herb itself contains dangerous substances called pyrrolizidine alkaloids that are highly toxic to the liver. In July 2001, the U.S. Food and Drug Administration required that all oral products containing comfrey be removed from the market. The United Kingdom, Australia, Canada, and Germany have also banned the sale of oral products containing comfrey. However, as pyrrolizidine alkaloids are absorbed through the skin as well as orally, a comfrey ointment should also not be used, as it may produce harmful amounts of these alkaloids in the body or enter the body directly through broken skin.

Symphytum officinale, though known as a "small" remedy because its mental and emotional picture is currently undeveloped, is homeopathically useful to stimulate the body to heal fractured bones and periosteum that are slow to repair. Though one would expect that comfrey, of which Symphytum officinale is a dilution, would produce toxic effects on bone, and thus on Essence, such is not the case. Although comfrey as yet sheds little light on causal stresses within Water, knowledge of its homeopathic properties in healing trauma fractures is well worth possessing.

HEARING DIMENSION ILLNESS: URINARY TRACT INFECTION

The biomedical diagnosis of urinary tract infection (UTI) can cover a host of acute and chronic genital and urinary tract symptoms including urgency to urinate, urinary frequency, dysuria, cramps and spasms of the bladder, itching or heat while urinating, nocturnal loss of urine, urethral discharge, general malaise, low-back or flank pain, nausea, vomiting, bladder tenderness, and chills. UTI is seen more frequently in women, who have shorter urethras than men have. Additionally, in men prostatic fluid acts as a shield against invasive bacteria.

In conventional medicine, the source of infection or inflammation is differentiated as to whether it occurs in the kidneys, bladder, urethra, prostate, or tubules attaching the testicles to the prostate. Thus, fever, malaise, nausea, and chills are seen with kidney and prostate infection. Urethral discharge is present with gonorrhea, chlamydia, and T-mycoplasma infections of the urethra, as opposed to typical bladder or kidney infections. Low-back and flank pain are associated with kidney (upper UT) infections. Nocturnal loss of urine may occur with any bladder infection, but it also results from some prostate infections. Interstitial cystitis, lacking a clearly infectious cause, is a problem all to itself.

It seems reasonable to accept at face value the conventional stance that UTIs relate solely to imperfect hygiene and bacteria successfully breaching urethral membrane and incubating in the bladder. Investigation, however, of at least one nonmechanical vulnerability that may precede the infection may shed further light on the problems of UTI and their Water-related issues. Awareness is useful, not only for treating, but also for preventing, UTIs.

In TCM, the Lower Warmer refers to a location in the body below the navel, especially encompassing the Kidney and Liver. In TCM diagnosis, Damp Heat in the Lower Warmer can present the symptoms described above and can also reflect, as well as engender, weakness of the Kidneys. The treatment principle in TCM involves clearing the Lower Warmer of Dampness and Heat, while also spreading Bladder Qi. Acupuncture treatments can be effective in accomplishing this and eliminating discomfort. From a nutritional standpoint one is also well-advised to avoid dampness-causing foods.

HEARING DIMENSION ILLNESS: URINARY TRACT INFECTION
HOMEOPATHIC REMEDY

Staphysagria

Staphysagria (stavesacre) individuals, in particular women, are unusually sensitive to rudeness and are deeply invested in a sense of honor; not surprisingly their self-esteem is often poor. They frequently have great difficulty confronting another individual and have developed an ingrained pattern of suppressing their indignation. Should they succeed in venting their considerable anger, they frequently pay for it with abdominal pain. They often have a strong libido, and sexuality can be prominent. Women who need the homeopathic remedy Staphysagria often have a history of UTIs stemming from early or frequent sexual activity. Their physical complaints can include severe cases of dental carries, especially during pregnancy, and stupefying headaches.

Staphysagria has a powerful affinity for the teeth, and the remedy is useful when the patient has had an extensive history of tooth decay. TCM teaches that the teeth are an extension of the bones, both consisting largely of calcium. If the bones represent our inner stability and worth, the teeth are their outwardly visual expression. A Staphysagria individual's vulnerability is understood as both reflecting and promoting a crumbling of inner worth, of which tooth decay is the physical evidence. The individual feels the presence of entropy closely, and this feeling contains destructive implications for the integrity of tissue such as the epithelium and bone. Our reading of the Staphysagria vulnerability reveals the centrality of supporting the patient's feeling of self-worth; this is accomplished when the patient is respected, and his sense of integrity as a person is allowed to remain intact.

Other remedies meriting use or study in relation to UTIs are Natrum phosphoricum and Mandragora officinarum.

HEARING DIMENSION ILLNESS: MÉNIÈRE'S DISEASE

Ménière's disease presents a derangement of the inner ear and vestibular system that can severely adversely affect hearing and balance. An individual may experience dizziness and tinnitus as well as progressive hearing loss, usually in one ear. Additionally, there can be numerous signs of Kidney deficiency: weariness, faintness, edema, and great sensitivity of the dorsal vertebrae. Whether it is a cause or a symptom of Ménière's disease, the volume and pressure of the endolymph of the inner ear apparently fluctuates.

A TCM modeling of how the endolymph might be altered in Ménière's disease would show that Phlegm is inhibiting the cleansing action of respiratory Qi. Phlegm clogging the upper Warmer, the anatomical area that includes the head and chest, would be found to cloud the senses. An acupuncture treatment protocol for Ménière's disease to clear Phlegm also addresses the symptom of lower vertebral sensitivity: In addition to clearing Phlegm, the treatment uses the Governing Vessel points of the lower dorsal spine as well as lateral points from the urinary bladder to tonify Kidney deficiency.

Because the eyes and skin, for example, may also be involved in Ménière's disease, the operation of the vestibular system in this disease might be extended into dimensions other than hearing. Yet, the ear is the opening of the Kidney, through which positional disorientation is disturbed. The ringing in the ear that frequently accompanies the vertigo in Ménière's disease manifests a deficiency of Kidney Essence, a finite substance whose depletion is associated with aging and entropy. This state of entropy not only pertains to Water, but may express a temporary relapse to a bygone time before the gill slits of a distant, marine ancestor evolved into our modern ears.

HEARING DIMENSION ILLNESS: MÉNIÈRE'S DISEASE
HOMEOPATHIC REMEDY

Chininum sulphuricum

Often employed to treat Ménière's disease, the remedy Chininum sulphuricum merits attention. This remedy comes into play when a patient feels enormously depleted, as, for example, following loss of blood, and suffers from vertigo and tinnitus. On the mental level the patient is excessively sensitive, has muddled thoughts, and fears of impending evil, or of what the future may hold. At its positive pole, the remedy state can manifest with buoyancy, clarity of mind, and a desire to make many plans.

Along with Selenium, the Chininum sulphuricum remedy pictures the price we pay when we become so depleted that we lose ground to entropy.

HEARING DIMENSION ILLNESS: CYSTIC FIBROSIS

More perfectly than any other condition, cystic fibrosis (CF) captures broad themes of Water. CF is a recessive, genetic, chronic disease involving the generalized dysfunction of the exocrine glands. CF affects multiple organ systems with increased viscosity of bronchial, pancreatic, and other mucous gland secretions and a consequent blockage of glandular ducts. People with CF have high levels of salt in their sweat, and the sweat test is the most common test for CF.[12] (Salty, according to TCM, is the flavor directly associated with the Kidney.) Most importantly, a thick, sticky mucous in the lungs produces persistent wheezing, a dry, unproductive, at times paroxysmal cough, shortness of breath, rapid breathing, and frequent lung infections. CF's gastrointestinal effects are experienced mostly in the intestines, pancreas, and liver. Pancreatic fibrosis—clogging of the organ's ducts and insufficiency of pancreatic enzymes—prevents the body from breaking down food and contributes to malabsorption, especially of fats, resulting in malnutrition. Half of the people born with CF die by 30 years of age, primarily from lung disease.[13]

As of 2002, according to data from the Cystic Fibrosis Foundation, about 30,000 Americans, 20,000 Europeans, and 3,000 Canadians have CF. In the U.S. the disease occurs mainly in Caucasians whose ancestors came from northern Europe, and it is therefore less common in African Americans, Native Americans, and Asian Americans. It is estimated that about 1 in every 20 Americans is an unaffected carrier of an abnormal CF gene and is unaware of being a carrier. Approximately 2,500 newborns in the U.S. are diagnosed with CF each year.[12,14,15]

Infertility resulting from CF largely affects men but also women. It is estimated that at least 97% of men with CF have absent vasa deferentia.[16] In women with CF, fertility difficulties can result from thickened cervical mucous and malnutrition that disrupts ovulation.[17]

In 1989, NIDDK-sponsored research teams at the University of Michigan and at the Hospital for Sick Children in Toronto, Canada, identified the gene responsible for CF and named its protein product "cystic fibrosis transmembrane conductance regulator" (CFTR). The gene was mapped to chromosome 7q.[12,15] In order to develop CF, a child must be born with two copies of the autosomal recessive gene, one from each parent. Although about 500 different mutations have been identified worldwide, the most common mutation, called delta F508, occurs in 70% of all defective CF genes; the CFTR protein it encodes is missing a single amino acid at position 508. CFTR levels are highest in the epithelial cells lining the inner surfaces of the pancreas, sweat and salivary glands, intestine, and reproductive organs. Normal CFTR protein serves as a channel transporting chloride ions out of the cells in which it is embedded. However, CF airway cells decrease secretion of chloride and increase absorption of sodium, which affects the flow of water: airway cells may thus absorb more water than normal, depleting mucus and other airway secretions of water, and making them thick and sticky.[15]

The intriguing question has always been, "Why do Caucasian populations, those of European descent, have an overwhelmingly higher frequency of CF than do other populations?" In fact, CF is the most fatal common autosomal recessive disorder among Caucasians. Attempts to answer this question have focused on speculation about what has been termed, "the heterozygote (carrier) advantage of the CF mutation"—that perhaps over thousands of years, the CF mutuation has offered protection against various other deadly diseases that have particularly plagued Europeans. Indeed, one study suggests that "haplotype data demonstrate that delta F508 occurred more than 52,000 years ago, in a population genetically distinct from any present European group, and spread throughout Europe in chronologically distinct expansions, which are responsible for the different frequencies of delta F508 in Europe."[18] CFTR's selective heterozygote advantages are theorized to include survival of chloride- and water-secreting diarrhea, cholera, malaria, and, especially concerning Europeans, who adopted a dairy-milk diet, resistance to lactose-caused diarrhea, while they were still lactose intolerant.[19,20,21]

The literature about CF, as well as my own practice, suggests that persons with CF are seldom depressed or bitter. Could they be imbued with a sense of the historical undercurrent of the disease? Could they, in genetic or karmic terms, carry within themselves the legacy and burden of having protected mankind against deadly diseases through dark times over hundreds of generations?

HEARING DIMENSION ILLNESS: CYSTIC FIBROSIS
HOMEOPATHIC REMEDY

Niccolum

Niccolum (made from nickel) has been found to be a useful remedy in treating CF. Its materia medica describes a haughty, high-achieving problem solver who is adept at suppressing his emotions, and who is alternately friendly and aggressive.

HEARING DIMENSION ILLNESS: LYME DISEASE

In the U.S., in 2008, the CDC reported 28,921 confirmed and 6,277 probable cases of Lyme disease, representing a 5% increase in confirmed cases compared to 2007.[22] These official figures, reported to the CDC by the state health departments, conceal serious contentions surrounding every aspect of Lyme disease, from the actual number of cases, the accuracy of the diagnosis and tests for the disease, the efficacy and safety of medications used to cure it, the range and durations of symptoms, the effectiveness of a Lyme disease vaccine, to whether or not the disease recurs or can persist indefinitely. Dr. C. Ben Beard, chief of the Bacterial Diseases Branch of the Division of Vector Borne Infectious Diseases at

CDC, states that studies over the last 20 years have indicated that underreporting has been a problem, and suggests that actually 3 to 12 times more cases occur than the number reported to the CDC.[23]

Lyme disease is caused by the spirochete bacterium *Borrelia burgdorferi* and is transmitted by the bite of an infected, miniscule deer tick. The CDC's 2008 case definition describes it as a disease with "protean manifestations, including dermatologic, rheumatologic, neurologic, and cardiac abnormalities."[24] Over a period of days to weeks in the beginning of the disease process, about 60% to 80% of patients develop a bullseye skin rash, called erythema migrans, which can be accompanied by other nonspecific symptoms, particularly fatigue, headache, fever, mood disturbances, joint pain, and muscle pain. Later manifestations can include joint swelling ending in chronic arthritis; meningitis; Bell's palsy; disorder of the spinal nerve roots and nerves, and rarely, inflammation of the brain and spinal cord; acute, but short-term atrioventricular blocks and inflammation of the heart muscles.[24] Beyond the complications described in the CDC's 2008 case definition, an extensive range of symptoms has been ascribed to Lyme disease, including neuropathies in various parts of the body, poor concentration and memory loss, blurred vision and eye pain, chest pain, and palpitations.[25]

Yet the diagnosis of Lyme disease by the two-tiered criteria of positive ELISA and western blot tests "fails to detect up to 90% of cases and does not distinguish between acute, chronic, or resolved infection."[25] Cases of chronic, persistent, recurrent, and refractory Lyme disease still go largely unrecognized, although new research within various disciplines is beginning to identify long-term manifestations, related strains, persistent symptoms after treatment, neuropsychiatric repercussions, and a propensity for relapse.[23,25] According to a 2004 report by The International Lyme and Associated Diseases Society, "There is no reliable, commercially available culture assay that can confirm the eradication of the organism. Using experimental techniques, however, *B. burgdorferi* has been detected in virtually every organ in the body, and the spirochete has a strong predilection for the central nervous system."[25]

In his presentation on "Immune Evasion Mechanisms of Pathogenic Spirochetes," Dr. Richard Marconi of Virginia Commonwealth University made the case that "Most spirochetal infections of humans can be chronic and in the absence of treatment can persist indefinitely."[23] Dr. Robert Dantzer of the University of Illinois at Urbana-Champaign concluded in his lecture "From Inflammation to Sickness Behavior: The Role of Cytokines," that "the initial inflammatory event from years earlier (due to infection or trauma) may be reactivated at a later point and, because of that past event, fail to turn off after being reactivated—causing chronic sickness symptoms."[23]

Available data show that antibiotics remain the treatment of choice in managing Lyme disease, but how large a dose to give, when and how, and for how long are still little understood, and the side effects of the antibiotics can be debilitating. In one study comparing the effects of intravenous antibiotics versus placebo to treat Lyme encephalopathy, the researchers found potentially serious side effects, including thrombi, systemic infections, allergic reactions, and gall bladder disease in 19% of patients receiving the IV antibiotic.[26]

Lyme Disease and TCM

In TCM, Lyme disease is classified under Kidney pathology. The pervasive weakening of the body under Lyme disease generally indicates a weakness of Kidney Yang. An effective immune response is lacking when it is needed, and the accumulation of persistent and similar infections, such as ehrlichiosis and babesiosis, erodes Kidney Yang. The current treatment that is overly reliant on antiobiotics and steroids and lacks a counterbalance to support the body's immune function also eventually weakens the Yang. The mental and emotional picture of fogginess and the sense that one's best effort are inadequate may consolidate into a self-perception of inadequacy that cascades: one feels inadequate because of inadequacy, weak because one is weak, and so on. Perhaps a TCM approach that bolsters the Kidney Yang while it addresses spirochetal infestation and inflammation may eventually complement the exclusively antibiotic treatment currently used in the West.

HEARING DIMENSION ILLNESS: LYME DISEASE
HOMEOPATHIC REMEDIES

Ledum and Lyme Nosode

Ledum is made from marsh tea, which can be found in bogs across northern Europe, Canada, and the U.S. Ledum is known to be effective as an important first-aid homeopathic remedy in treating ailments from insect bites. It helps to prevent infection and is also given for rheumatic pain and stiff, painful joints.

Ledum in combination with a nosode made from the Lyme disease infection may prove to be useful in treating Lyme disease. A nosode is prepared from diseased tissue such as bacteria, fungi, ova, parasites, virus particles, excretions, or secretions. Homeopathic nosodes can stimulate the body's immune system in response to a disease and help eliminate the pathogens naturally.

HEARING DIMENSION ILLNESS: SYPHILIS

Yet another spirochete, *Treponema pallidum* subspecies *pallidum*, which is the cause of syphilis, has a curious and controversial medical history. Other bacteria in the same genus cause yaws and bejel, transmitted through skin-to-skin contact or by drinking from the same glass. Research suggests that syphilis was first present in the New World, about 1,600 years ago—perhaps as a mutation of yaws, which evidence shows occurred in the New World at least 6,000 years ago—and is believed to have been brought to the Old World by Christopher Columbus and his crew.[27] The first recorded epidemic of syphilis in Europe broke out in 1495.[28]

Because of its numerous manifestations, syphilis, like Lyme disease, can masquerade as other conditions. Left to progress on its own through three developmental stages, syphilis illustrates the consolidating and self-perpetuating tendency of Water. From a TCM standpoint, it is apparent that syphilis most directly impairs the Kidneys.

In the first or primary stage of syphilis, one or more sores, or chancres, appear at the site where syphilis initially enters the body. These are usually firm, round, and painless, and remain visible for between three and six weeks. Left untreated, the infection may progress to the secondary stage, when one or several rashes replace the fading chancres. Although—even without treatment—these often clear up on their own, other symptoms may appear that include swollen lymph glands, fever, sore throat, hair loss, headaches, aching muscles, and fatigue. Late-stage or tertiary syphilis appears after the secondary-stage symptoms vanish, even if no ill effects are immediately noticed. This late stage includes damage to the internal organs, brain, nerves, eyes, heart, blood vessels, liver, bones, and joints. Paralysis, blindness, and dementia, which can eventually lead to death, may follow.

Data from the CDC show that from 2004 to 2008 the rate of primary and secondary syphilis in the U.S. rose from 2.7 to 4.5 per 100,000 population.[29] The highest rates in 2008 were reported in the South, in urban areas, among African-

Americans, and, most particularly, among men who have sex with men (MSM).

In 2008, 63% of all primary- and secondary-stage (P&S) syphilis cases in the U.S. were reported to be among MSM; these cases have been characterized by high rates of HIV comorbidity and high-risk sexual behaviors.[30]

According to the CDC, "Race and ethnicity in the United States are risk markers that correlate with other more fundamental determinants of health status such as poverty, access to quality health care. . . illicit drug use, and living in communities with high prevalence of STDs."[31]

Syphilis, Antibiotics, and TCM

Despite its powerful short-term effects, conventional treatment with antibiotics may also contribute to the consolidation and self-perpetuation of syphilis, many of whose manifold symptoms are passed on from generation to generation. One of TCM's greatest teachings is that it is insufficient to address only the pathogenic cause of disease; longer-lasting results are produced when the constitution is also supported, although clearly, in this case, the results may be less immediately dramatic than those of penicillin. TCM treatment appears to target the spirochete while it also supports the constitution's battle against the bacterium's deep and persistently harmful effects.

Overreliance on the antibiotic penicillin wins a battle but loses a war. Deprived of an opportunity to repel the syphilitic *Treponema* spirochete on its own, the body remains expectant of further assault and expends metabolic energy assembling a vigilant antibody force. The effort compromises immunity to syphilis, leaving the body susceptible to reinfection. The continuous presence within the body of an antibody force while no pathogen is present both resembles and promotes pathogenic autoimmunity. Thus, a weakness engendering a state of preparedness that includes susceptibility to despair, to dementia, or to an autoimmune condition, consolidates and imprints itself onto the Yang or DNA.

Before penicillin was discovered, the chief mode of treating syphilis in the West was a prescription of either arsenic or mercury. Mercury, in particular, made sense to physicians of the time because its toxicological effects so closely resemble syphilitic symptoms. Doctors in those days intuitively, if not explicitly, acquiesced to homeopathic reasoning with regard to homeopathy's basic Law of Similars. Of course, when biomedical physicians began to utilize mercury, they gave far too much of it, thereby creating a genuinely toxicological reaction in patients.

TCM theory also encompasses homeopathy, and arsenic oxide has been applied in TCM for more than 500 years, based on TCM's principle of "using a toxic agent against a toxic agent."[32]

A madness is often found in the despair of individuals with late-stage syphilis, a madness that consists of furious circular reasoning. Its manifestation, which also persists among descendants of those infected, expresses the following radical disjunct: A purely sexual response to hardship fuels a cycle in which the entropy one tries to avoid returns, redoubled in strength.

Syphilitic remedies indispensable to any homeopathic study include the nosode Syphilinum and Mercurius (quicksilver).

THE HEARING DIMENSION: PERSONAL THERAPEUTIC PRACTICES AND MASTERS OF EXPRESSION

In addition to treatment within TCM, homeopathy, and biomedicine, a number of therapeutic practices may promote health within the sense dimension of hearing. **Table 1** reviews some of these practices.

Table 2 on the following page lists a few Masters throughout history who have exemplified either the positive or negative poles of the sense dimension of hearing by strongly expressing one of the sides of the consolidation-entropy axis, the core issue of the hearing dimension.

Table 1. Hearing Dimension: Health-promoting Practices

Be moderate in all things	**Maintain good body heat**
Secure your family's safety and security	**Find and fulfill your life's meaning and mission**
Improve your community	**Consider and secure your legacy**
Nurture the mother of hearing, *Smell*: "Strive to remain centered"	

Table 2. Examples of Masters of the Sense Dimension of Hearing

NEGATIVE POLE: ENTROPY	POSITIVE POLE: CONSOLIDATION
Edwin Hubble: the expanding universe	Carl Gustav Jung: the collective unconscious
Sándor Ferenczi: (*The Unwanted Child and the Death Instinct*)	Hindu teachers of reincarnation
	Bert Hellinger, cofounder of Constellation Therapy

CHAPTER SEVEN

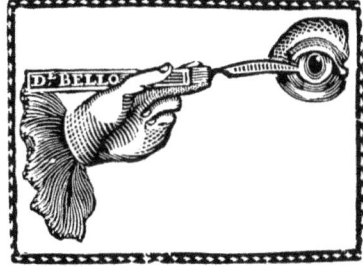

THE DIMENSION OF SIGHT

THE SENSE DIMENSION OF SIGHT

PHASE	WOOD
ORGAN	LIVER
CORE ISSUE	CREATIVITY–CHAOS

Sight instantaneously interprets the chaos of light into brilliant, creative, and meaningful images. Through sight, we are not passive viewers of a completed world of objects. We are, rather, active participants, meeting the world and constructing interpretations that take light into account. The act of vision is fundamentally creative, imposing order and fitting patterns on the chaos of photons. To see is to create.

The complexity and ambiguity of visual stimuli are irritatingly dangerous. If we fail to compose relevant images, we find ourselves prey to predators, potholes, or onrushing traffic. With every shift in our visual field, with every new irritation of our optic neural cells, we are called upon to react and to creatively transform that irritation into meaningful images. The inability to make clear distinctions and clean decisions can leave us paralyzed and resentful as we try to accommodate opposing notions simultaneously.

Relevant and meaningful images are grounded in the light of nature. Ungrounded creativity (delusion, fantasy, hallucination) is an invitation to descend into chaos. Yet, when our vision is not sufficiently creative, we impose constraints and galling limitations on ourselves that obscure the beckoning light of our own liberty.

The emotional reaction to constraint is anger, even when we have self-imposed the constraint. Anger turned inward on the self can manifest as depression. When anger is overwhelming, we may lose insight/sight. Commitment to anger forfeits all possibility of creative response. Resolution of anger involves recovering unseen possibilities, re-envisioning our situation, seeing matters in a new light. We choose between chaos and anger or the grounded liberation of insight.

Sight is profoundly linked with insight. When we see the light, see the truth, we are set free. But vision is a panoramic sense; like Adam and Eve, by taking everything in, we too are at risk of seeing too much, of taking on greater knowledge than we can handle. Thankfully, we need not be like King Lear, who acquired insight only after becoming blind. Sightlessness, therefore, is another door to chaos.

Possibly, however, no one is ever truly and completely blind: blindsight, the ability to perceive elements of the environment even when the brain's visual lobes do not function, was confirmed, in 2008, in a report by a team of international researchers of a patient with bilateral damage to the primary visual (striate) cortex who navigated around numerous barriers placed along a long corridor.[1] The ability to see nonvisually reflects the firing of neurons located deep in the midbrain where subconscious activation promotes intuition-like awareness. Because not only the eye, but also the entire body appears to respond visually, healthy vision might be conceived as the appropriate, but also creative, interpretation of photons. More than any other sense, seeing grants us possibilities and freedom.

THE LIVER IN TRADITIONAL CHINESE MEDICINE

The Liver in TCM is posited to be the storehouse of blood. Its healthy influence sustains the smooth and even movement of Qi and also rules over the contractile aspects of the tendons. From a biomedical perspective, we would consider these functions to be essentially neurological. When the liver is dysfunctional, digestive and bile-related disturbances, as well as menstrual problems and spasms or tremors in the muscles, can occur. Eye disorders are often considered liver-related. At the emotional level, anger, indecisiveness, stagnation, and depression can result.

In TCM, the Liver and its paired organ, the Gall Bladder, belong to the Phase of Wood. Wood is associated with Wind, whether external (environmental) or internal. This implies a presentation of symptoms that have a rising or upwelling quality and the potential to change rapidly.

The Liver is the residence of the Hun, the Ethereal Soul. Though it inhabits the blood, the Hun is said to survive the body at death. The Hun influences visions, dreams, and the creative well of the unconscious.

In TCM, symptoms of Liver disharmonies include depression, anger, irritability, belching, nausea, vomiting, abdominal pain, menstrual problems, dizziness, tremors, spasms, headaches, hypertension, eye problems, and liver diseases.

SIGHT DIMENSION CORE ISSUE: THE CREATIVITY–CHAOS AXIS

Of all the organs, the liver is the most creative in terms of its ability to regenerate. Lose the function of the majority of the liver, and it may rebound and rebuild. But its creative powers do not end there.

The lobes of the liver are composed primarily of hepatocytes. These cells conduct a remarkable range of complex and vital tasks without further specialization. This implies that there is a capacity for decisions to be made at cellular and organ levels. The metabolic engine of the liver synthesizes (creates) the plasma proteins used in blood clotting as well as in anticoagulents, bile acids, growth hormones, and steroid hormones. These same liver cells remove metabolic wastes and exogenous toxins, neutralizing them in preparation for excretion. The cells also process the nutrients absorbed into the blood through digestion. They store sugars, fats, vitamins, and minerals, releasing them when levels in the blood are low. The liver has immune functions mediated by phagocytes, a different type of cell.

CREATIVITY

The sense dimension of sight provides the experiential example that guides all other human creative impulses and endeavors. In health, sight is intrinsically creative within limits; it is decisive, discerning, and liberating. Consistent with the Liver's role in the promotion of flow, the creative aspect of sight originates neither in the ego nor in the will, nor does it manifest harshly. Creativity rather embodies Keats's expression, "Beauty is truth, truth beauty." Creative action at its best represents purity of vision and global awareness of possibilities. The greatest examples of creativity—such as those found in Shakespeare's writings—are suffused with compassion.

We cannot assume that our sensitivities are entirely inborn. Sensitivity to the nuances of music, to a great painting, to the suffering of others, can be cultivated. To a certain extent, our sensitivity to the spread of microbes or to possible dangers in air travel can also be modified. Unless the capability to influence sensitivity exists, inner knowledge has scant value with regard to health. Susceptibility to illness is rooted within the tenor of our thoughts and in the quality of our choices. Mental hygiene is critical, because whether our dreams are nightmares or visions of glory, they have a tendency to influence the tenor of our lives.

The specific quality of an individual's sensitivity is a source of diagnostic information. Consequently, a shift in sensitivity, whether it be for better or for worse, is a momentous event. Independent of treatment, an individual's sensitivity and his ability to heal are inseparable.

It is a common conceit that creativity is principally a human mental capacity. But creativity occurs at all levels and in all animate and inanimate systems.

CHAOS

In Greek mythology, *Khaos*, or Chaos, was conceived to be the first of the primeval gods, the void of infinite space out of which everything in creation was formed. According to Ovid, Chaos was a confused mass containing the elements of all created things. Chaos personified the abyss or unformed matter, the opposite of birth and creativity on the creativity-chaos axis, the core issue in the dimension of sight.[2]

Chaos may be approached through indecision, delusion, anger, or through being visually, cognitively, or spiritually overwhelmed. These traits of chaos are major gateways to the stagnation of Liver Qi, and they imply the existence of different disorders and different remedy states.

The failure to resolve chaos and to see hidden yet vital creative options sets the energetic stage for a number of chronic illnesses. Setting the stage may consist of a decades-long process of minor decrements and compromises in thought, deed, and vision. This accretion of ills tends to be invisible, so that the trail there and back is obscured.

Recognizing chaos and seeking remedies are remarkable, creative steps. Chaos is not a disease or a biomedical disorder, and thus it may be lightly dismissed in error. To arrive at the recognition of the corrosiveness of chaos in its several guises is to have already approached healing

SIGHT DIMENSION: CHRONIC ILLNESSES

SIGHT DIMENSION ILLNESS: EYE INFLAMMATION

Although eye inflammations mainly tend to be acute, at times chronic symptoms, such as drusen, do crop up. Drusen are fatty deposits on the retina that can develop into macular degeneration, corneal ulcers, and persistent allergies, causing burning, smarting, swelling, lachrimation, and granulation. Soft drusen are associated with loss of vision.

SIGHT DIMENSION ILLNESS: EYE INFLAMMATION
HOMEOPATHIC REMEDY

Euphrasia

Euphrasia (also known as eyebright) is one of the major remedies to consider for either acute eye inflammation or chronic symptoms, such as drusen. Eyebright's history as an herb that enhances inner vision and awareness is reflected in the homeopathic remedy's mental and emotional picture that predisposes or reflects the desire to see, but also has difficulty seeing things as they genuinely are. The presence of this mind-set is evident from the appearance of confusion, amelioration of symptoms by face-washing, a sense of darkness, and a variety of delusions.

One of my patients, who presented with severe allergies, inflamed conjunctiva, and drusen, stated that she realized the symptoms arose after she constantly denied that her living room was outmoded. She came to me when she suddenly understood how badly the space needed to be remodeled; the flash of insight fueled an impetus to undertake both the project and treatment, which also improved her symptoms.

SIGHT DIMENSION ILLNESS: SEIZURE DISORDERS

Individuals suffering from seizure disorders or epilepsy are prone to experiencing an electrical storm of neural firing within the brain's circuitry. In TCM, the condition relates to the element Wood and the dimension of sight for two main reasons: the fluttery tremors and rapidly changing features of convulsive activity conform to TCM's diagnostic category of Wind, or, in line with our current analysis, with chaos; and the clonic features of convulsions, meaning their violent muscular contractions, relate to the function of the Liver, said to govern the action of the tendons.

SIGHT DIMENSION ILLNESS: SEIZURE DISORDERS
HOMEOPATHIC REMEDIES

Cuprum metallicum and Zincum metallicum, two of the homeopathic remedies indicated for seizure disorders, demonstrate Yang within Yin, a relationship between the suppression of emotions and convulsive activity, which in TCM may be classified as Internal Liver Wind. At the opposite extreme, two other seizure-disorder remedies, Agaricus muscarius and Cicuta virosa, demonstrate Yin within Yang, a relationship between excessive stimulation and deficiency-based, convulsive activities.

Cuprum metallicum

Unable to allow a free flow of emotion because they find it disturbing, persons in need of Cuprum metallicum, made from copper, suppress and transmute their feelings. Their need for inner control generates a powerful work ethic, a venting of emotions through irascibility, and a tendency to mimic others or perform antics. Emotionally cramped, they are also subject to external, muscular cramping. The Cuprum metallicum person is driven by an attitude toward authority that betrays the remedy's radical disjunct: excessive respect for authority invites an ambitious need to overcome and transcend authority. Because muscular cramps and spasms lie on a continuum with convulsive activity, Cuprum metallicum may be an effective treatment for some types of seizures.

Zincum metallicum

Although it certainly also manifests on its own terms, Zincum metallicum often follows well after Cuprum metallicum. As one might expect, an individual moving on from Cuprum metallicum to Zinc metallicum is not only less emotionally cramped, but also has improved rather than worsened by a discharge of anger. His inner control, instead of expressing a response to the massive oppressiveness of authority, has been reduced to a superego issue that provides us with Zircum metallicum's radical disjunct, possibly resolvable by therapy: excessive acceptance of the authority of a productive father invites resistance to one's own productivity.

The Zincum metallicum individual, although also emotionally shut down, suffers from a social phobia and an inability to cast off even the smallest of disappointments. He is likely to be more helpful to others than to himself. Prone to anger and to a nonproductive discharge of nervous energy, he is subject to mental burnout, spasms, twitching, and convulsions, for which Zincum metallicum can be an effective treatment.

Agaricus muscarius (Amanita)

This remedy is made from an intoxicating and neurologically agitating fungus called toad stool, fly agaric, or bug agaric. This fungus contains several toxic compounds, the best known of which is muscarin. Its chaotic effects include a distorted sense of perspective, lack of restraint, and superhuman physical strength. Persons in need of Agaricus muscarius can have an unusual interest in bizarre subjects and strong fears in relation to their health. They may exhibit chorea and all manner of involuntary and excessively expressive movements. These lie on a continuum of convulsive activity that includes twitching, spasms, and epilepsy.

The remedy's radical disjunct can be expressed in terms of an excess of reactivity that invites dullness. The Agaricus muscarius state manifests reactivity so excessively that the vital force is compelled to balance the exaltation with its opposite emotion, a sense of detachment. The remedy's materia medica includes delusions that one's arm and legs do not belong to oneself and that something foreign is alive in one's head. Convulsions and other features related to the remedy-state imbalance are redressed by a constitutional dose of Agaricus muscarius.

Cicuta virosa

This remedy, made from water hemlock, also manifests an excess of reactivity that invites dullness. Its radical disjunct is similar to that of Agaricus muscarius, the difference being that Cicuta virosa's excess of reactivity and lack of balance are expressed in terms that more narrowly relate to a distortion of perspective and a sense that objects are either too close or too distant. The Cicuta virosa individual is also excessively naïve and may think and behave like a child. At its deficient, opposite pole, which is responsible for its convulsive activity, the remedy features a tendency to stare blankly, distrust others, and experience oneself as estranged from society. Cicuta virosa is a major remedy to think of when treating convulsions resulting from fright or an injury to the brain, or a grand mal seizure—currently called a tonic-clonic seizure—that features a loss of consciousness and violent muscle contractions.

SIGHT DIMENSION ILLNESS: VASCULAR HEADACHES

Vascular headaches are diagnosed in TCM as manifesting disharmony of Liver Yang. Disappointment, resentment, or suppressed anger is viewed as a constraint on the Liver's energy. As a result, the general free flow of bodily energy, or Qi, is impeded, and Liver blood is reined in. The metaphor of a compost heap usefully conveys the state of stagnation and generation of internal Heat that follows. Its beginning manifestation, termed hyperactive Liver Yang in TCM, is accurately mirrored in the materia medica of the homeopathic remedy Iris versicolor. A subsequent, and more extreme manifestation, termed Liver Fire Rising, is reproduced by the materia medica of homeopathic Sanguinaria.

SIGHT DIMENSION ILLNESS: VASCULAR HEADACHES
HOMEOPATHIC REMEDIES

Iris versicolor: "Conscience of the Public"

Individuals in need of Iris versicolor, made from a perennial herb known as blue flag (and interestingly, also called liver lily), suffer from vascular headaches that occur in a context of nervousness and irritability. This hyperactive Liver Yang remedy state can also include visual disturbances, hypoglycemia, a sour stomach, and pustular skin discharges. In its exalted expression, an Iris versicolor individual is hardly at all lily-livered; in fact, he is likely to laugh about his own fears for his health. The irritability and sensitivity of Iris versicolor has an affinity with taking a stand about publicly outrageous issues (the remedy can remind us of Kali carbonicum's moral intolerance). This gives us the remedy's radical disjunct: excessive sensitivity to criticism promotes one's own censoriousness.

Sanguinaria

The remedy Sanguinaria, made from an herbaceous perennial known as bloodroot, is indicated for headaches caused by more dynamic consequences of constriction of the blood capillaries than those seen in Iris versicolor. Sanguinaria's upward surge of Heat caused by the rising of Liver Fire generates not only severe headaches and dim vision, but also the chaos of alternating symptoms, dry and burning sensations, and a stupefying sensitivity to sound. The remedy state can generate a hectic flush of red, blotchy skin eruptions, metrorrhagia (Reckless Blood in TCM), and a very nearly cataleptic state of confusion. The remedy's central issue, which can be seen as a ramping up of Iris versicolor's reaction to criticism, is a sensitivity to insult sufficient to produce rage. The radical disjunct: an excessive reaction to provocation invites its opposite, stupefaction.

SIGHT DIMENSION ILLNESS: CLUSTER HEADACHES

A cluster headache (also known as migrainous neuralgia) is not life-threatening, but can be so painful that the sufferer may consider suicide or engage in head-banging to stop it. Cluster headaches are one-sided, more common in men than in women, and occur in cyclical patterns, or cluster periods that may occur daily for months, followed by remission periods when the headache attacks stop completely. Scientists do not know what causes cluster headaches, but they appear to be associated with a sudden release of serotonin or histamine.[3]

Although the materia medica of the remedy Spigelia cannot explain why cluster headaches occur, it may shed some light on their meaning.

SIGHT DIMENSION ILLNESS: CLUSTER HEADACHES
HOMEOPATHIC REMEDY

Spigelia: "Looking Daggers at Me"

Spigelia, made from demarara pinkroot, also known as wormgrass, demonstrates the liability associated with seeing and knowing too much. Spigelia is of singular importance not only for cluster headaches, but for violent and radiating pain generally. Its migraine headaches arise in the occiput or neck, from where they tend to settle in or over the left eye. Individuals needing Spigelia appear to develop their ailments after quarrels; when breathing too deeply they often become anxious. They also worry excessively about their relatives, and are prone to cursing.

The remedy's most striking feature is its sensitivity to sharp objects, as a result of which a person greatly fears anything that happens to be jagged, pointed, or brittle. He is excessively sensitive to touch, and his pains suggest to him that he has been stabbed or threatened with stabbing. The eyes (by means of which the sharpness of objects is perceived) feel not only terribly painful, but also too large. The eyes may also feel as if they are being pushed forward or backwards deep into their sockets. The remedy state features palpitations and violent, sharp chest pains that one may conjecture reflect a fear of being stabbed in the heart. Spigelia's radical disjunct may be expressed as follows: an enlarged perception of danger invites its opposite, awareness of pinpoint and pinprick hazards.

SIGHT DIMENSION ILLNESS:
COMPLEX REGIONAL PAIN SYNDROME

Complex regional pain syndrome (CRPS) is a chronic condition previously called reflex sympathetic dystrophy and causalgia. As yet, little is known about the causes of CRPS, and few treatments have been effective. There is no clear evidence that genetic factors play a role in its development, which is more common in women and with increasing age. CRPS most often affects the arms, legs, hands, or feet after some sort of trauma, even a minimal one, the most common being surgery, sprains, fractures, and crushing. The key symptom of CRPS is intense, continuous pain that is far out of proportion to the severity of the injury.[4] The pain can be intolerable, violent, and wildly distracting in response to even minimal levels of nerve stimulation.

Because so little about CRPS is understood, many previously assumed (and some still do) that the condition was purely psychogenic, but it is now generally believed that some nerve trauma may trigger the cascade of events leading to CRPS.[4] In one pivotal study, in 2006, skin biopsies showed an up to 29% reduction in nerve fibers in affected tissue.[5] The study authors concluded that damage to the nerves of the skin produced CRPS.

Because there is no cure for CRPS, biomedical treatment is targeted at relieving pain. Besides physical therapy and psychotherapy, which helps deal with the profound effects of the sometimes unremitting and crippling pain, treatment can involve use of topical analgesics; antiseizure drugs, antidepressants, corticosteroids, and opioids; surgical interventions; intravenous administration of phentolamine; and intrathecal drug pumps that inject opioids and anesthetic agents into the spinal fluid.[6] Because patients with CRPS are unlikely to see a homeopathic practitioner until they have exhausted every means possible to relieve their pain with conventional treatments, homeopaths generally see these patients when they are at the end of their rope and have compromised their life force. Had they come to a homeopath before this, at least one homeopathic remedy, Hypericum, might have been of benefit to them.

SIGHT DIMENSION ILLNESS:
COMPLEX REGIONAL PAIN SYNDROME
HOMEOPATHIC REMEDY

Hypericum perforatum

The substance from which this remedy, Hypericum, is made is familiar to us as a popular herbal antidepressant, St. John's wort, or hypericum perforatum. The common name St. John's wort is thought to be derived from the time when the plant blooms, around the 24th of June, the date on which John the Baptist is supposed to have been beheaded. Recent interest in St. John's Wort has grown because of its action as an antiviral agent and its potential therapeutic use, currently under investigation, for treatment of cancer.

Insofar as it successfully buttresses a debilitative nervous system, St. John's wort is an effective mood enhancer. Yet when St. John's wort is highly diluted homeopathically, it addresses symptoms of an overstimulated and inflamed nervous system.

Hypericin, the active agent found in the plant, is considered responsible for the inhibition of the enzyme system known as monoamine oxidase (MAO). Hypericin is known to be toxic to most animals because of its photooxidative properties: in fact, hypericism is a state of skin sensitivity induced by visible light, caused by the ingestion of hypericin-containing plants and feed. With hypericin's presence in the body, numerous compounds found in foods and drugs fail to be oxidized. Also, hypericin interacts with tyramine-containing substances such as alcohol, narcotics, yeasts, and certain foods. Research suggests that hypericin's radical disjunct is derived from its two opposing effects: its actions associated with depression, but conversely also with providing motivational impetus.

An individual able to benefit from a constitutional dose of Hypericum may, under the right circumstances, prove susceptible to developing CRPS. Such a person possesses an overly strong nervous system, which is to say he reacts to normal levels of stimulation with preternatural speed and acuity. He is also prone to feel nervous and hurried, a state of mind that can devolve into tearful melancholy conjoint with the avoidance of pain. Polarity within the remedy state also encompasses two distinctive mental features: an exalted sensation that he is raised high up in the air; and also its opposite, a melancholy belief that a part of him has been repudiated by God and is, therefore, split off from his being.

St. John's wort's historical use in spiritual practice may help define these symptoms. The Greek word, hyper meaning "above" denotes exaltation, while the Greek for eikon, means "picture." Hyper-eikon alludes to an ancient belief that when the plant is hung above a picture it summons down to earth an ability to ward off evil spirits.

Electrons operate within electrical devices and in human cells alike. Hypericum's radical disjunct gives a literal meaning to an electrical metaphor: Hypericum's exalted state carries excessive voltage, but in the absence of a grounding wire Hypericum invites an electrical short-out and consequent scorching of the wires. Insofar as it assists an individual to become grounded, an appropriate dosage with Hypericum can act to alleviate the spiritual disconnect, neurological chaos, and hellish pain of CRPS.

SIGHT DIMENSION ILLNESS:
MODERN-DAY HYSTERIA

The word hysteria is derived from "hystera," Greek for uterus. From the time of the ancient Greeks until well into the 20th century, hysteria was seen as a woman's disease and believed, at various times, to reflect a sexually starved or retreating uterus; demon-possession; excessive religious fervor; seizures, fits, and manic behavior, stemming largely from repressed sexual desire; and imaginary fears and physical disorders. Fortunately, today, this prejudicial notion of hysteria has been largely discarded, and the word "hysteria" is currently used as a diagnosis only in France.

In the DSM-IV, published by the American Psychiatric Association, in 1994, the earlier label of "hysteria" has been replaced by "Dissociative (Conversion) Disorder" and "Conversion Disorder," terms describing motor and sensory symptoms, such as paralysis, pain, fits, dissociative identity, and depersonalization, which lack an observed neurological explanation, which are not feigned, and for which a psychosocial explanation can be given.

Indeed, the entire disorder is currently so little understood medically that it has also been given various other names such as "psychogenic," "somatization," "medically unexplained," "nonorganic"and "functional weakness," among others.[7] The disorder has been further broken down into subsets of symptoms, none of which can be explained by a general medical condition, a physical or laboratory investigation, or by substance use, including medications and drug abuse, and are considered by physicians to have a psychological, or inorganic, cause instead of a biological one: among others, these can be gastrointestinal symptoms, such as difficulty swallowing and irritable bowel syndrome; sexual symptoms, including lack or excess of sexual desire, erectile dysfunction, irregular menses, and vomiting throughout pregnancy; pseudoneurological symptoms, such as impaired balance, paralyzed muscles, collapsing weakness, fits, double vision, blindness, seizures, amnesia, and loss of consciousness; chronic fatigue syndrome; and hypochondria.

That a lack of a medical diagnosis for these symptoms is fairly common has been supported by a study, reported in 2000, of a cohort of 300 outpatients of a regional neurology clinic in Lothian, Scotland. The study's authors found that approximately one-third of new referrals at the clinic had neurological symptoms for which the physicians found no underlying, identifiable organic disease.[8]

Very little progress has been made in identifying the neurobiological mechanisms of conversion disorders. The work of Vuilleumier in the U.K. indicates that brain-imaging techniques have shown selective reductions in various cortices of the brain.[9] In one study report, in 2001, Vuilleumier and colleagues suggested that "hysterical conversion deficits may entail a functional disorder in striato-thalamocortical circuits controlling sensorimotor function and voluntary motor behaviour. . . ." The researchers concluded that "While hysterical disorders are usually defined by exclusion of an organic disease, the present findings of specific neurophysical correlates may. . . . help to reassure both patients and medical carers that hysterical symptoms are indeed functional, but nonetheless real, rather than mere imagination or malingering. . . .These findings provide novel constraints for a modern psychological theory of hysteria."[10]

The authors of this study concluded their report with a captivating quote from the great philosopher and psychologist William James in his series of Lowell lectures delivered, in 1896, to an audience of 900 ordinary Bostonians at a hall on Huntington Avenue, in Boston. James said from this podium: "Poor hysterics. First they were treated as victims of sexual trouble . . . then of moral perversity and mediocrity . . . then of imagination. Among the various rehabilitations which our age has seen, none are more deserving or humane. It is a real disease, but a mental disease."

SIGHT DIMENSION ILLNESS:
MODERN-DAY HYSTERIA
HOMEOPATHIC REMEDIES

The materia medica of homeopathic remedies described here will cover the remedy states of "hysterical grief." For the homeopath, hysteria, in general, reflects a generic radical disjunct to the effect that if one is excessively grounded in a particular worry one invites an ungrounded state of exaltation. When hysteria results from grief and suppressed anger, reliably held mental distinctions go by the wayside, and involuntary illogical thoughts and behaviors are promoted.

Ignatia: "Grief From Loss and Disappointment"

Ignatia is the most famous of all grief remedies in homeopathy. The Ignatia remedy state features silent grief, disappointment, outbursts of bitter anger, and shame. An individual needing this remedy is often self-contradictory, changeable, and dramatic. On the physical plane, a person may experience muscular spasms, a peculiar sensation like that of having a plum pit caught in the throat, a strong sensitivity to odors, headaches, and a changeable appetite. Frequently she will yawn and sigh.

If a woman is constitutionally predisposed to Ignatia, she will possess high ideals and expectations of the world. She will be deeply invested in the idea that the world is ruled by the principle that everything works out for the best. When a person with this belief suffers a loss, disappointment, or setback, and is incapable of jettisoning the idea of the ruling principle, the commitment to the ruling principle is clung to, but it diverts to its opposite: now the Ignatia client is invested in the idea that *nothing* works out for the best. The remedy's radical disjunct that everything always works out for the best invites a mirror-image certainty that everything works out for the worst; thus the Ignatia individual draws one victimization scenario after another to herself.

The Ignatia individual is so predisposed to disappointment, yet also, so hotly reactive that she quickly provokes the giver of even the most well-meaning comment into making an angry counter-retort. Thus, her interactions consistently spiral into arguments. Dumbfounded as to why this is so, she experiences herself as surrounded by rude and ill-meaning individuals. No other remedy so poignantly proves the adage that one makes one's own reality. It is wondrous to hear an Ignatia patient return to her practitioner after treatment and report, "I don't know why or how, but everyone is suddenly being nice to me."

Lilium tigranum: "Grief From Discord"

In homeopathy, the grief-related disordering of Liver Qi in Lilium tigranum, made from the well-known tiger lily, evokes both an exalted and hysterical response. Lilium tigranum's exaltation manifests in a person as an exaggerated sense of her importance; at the same time, she appears to be haughty, humorless, ungrateful, hurried, and irritable. A distraught state can emerge if discord undermines fulfillment in marriage and produces sexual guilt. If chaos then results, religious idealism, industriousness, and concern for business affairs can commingle with feelings of going crazy and violence.

On the physical plane, the remedy state includes palpitations, burning sensations in the palms of the hands and soles of the feet, a bearing-down sensation from the shoulders, thorax, left breast, or epigastrium into the pelvic region.[11] Lilium tigranum's radical disjunct might be straight out of Freud: suppression of sexual energy invites the return of sexual energy.

Berberis vulgaris: "Grief From a Hidden Wound"

Berberis vulgaris expresses hysteria that is the opposite of exaltation: a taciturn and inwardly-directed hysteria that features melancholy and an inability to think clearly. On the physical plane the remedy picture includes chilliness, radiating pains, dryness of the mucous membranes, and dirty brown pigmentation of the skin.

The trauma of Berberis vulgaris is that of a hidden wound; for example, a wound carried deep within from sexual abuse occurring in childhood, a wound to which its victim cannot demonstrably or directly respond. A hidden wound like this can also result if a woman ceases to be found sexually desirable by her husband once she has become a mother.

Berberis vulgaris is made from barberry, a shrub with gray, thorny branches that can grow to about nine feet tall. The thorny branches of barberry objectify a "Leave me alone" as opposed to a "You had better watch out" mind-set. The remedy state produces symptoms that reflect inward compression of anger and fear, and the target is most especially the kidney, bladder, and gall bladder stones. The radical disjunct of Berberis vulgaris: if you hide and consolidate a wound to the hardness of a stone, you invite its external exposure or expulsion.

Raphanus: "Grief From Irreconcilable Emotions"

Although it is possible to hold two completely opposite thoughts simultaneously within one's mind, it usually happens with a heavy price to pay. Made from a radish, the Raphanus remedy vividly pictures the degree to which sexual frustration and guilt experienced together can disorder Liver Qi. The hysteria of Raphanus presents a formidable challenge to logic and provides a perverse radical disjunct: sexual mania in a heterosexual man or woman invites revulsion for the opposite sex.

The Raphanus mind-set may either create or reflect havoc with the Liver's ability to manage the patency of energy. Liver Qi stagnates massively, but before this Qi has a chance to turn into Heat, it strikes out in a lateral direction (according to TCM, it invades the stomach), causing abdominal and epigastric pain, tightness of the chest, nausea, and excessive flatulence. Sleep is severely disordered by restlessness, distressing dreams, erethism (sexual excitability), and early morning waking.

A case from my files in which Raphanus was found to work beautifully provides some insight into its picture: My patient, a man in his early fifties, had been happily married to his wife for 17 years. Approximately four years earlier, she had fallen into a depression and began to experience a mental decline sufficiently severe as to gradually erode the foundation for their relationship. My patient described that, while caring for her, he grew debilitated from constantly cycling between hope for his marriage and despair of its ever being salvageable. When he came to see me he had finally decided that the marriage was completely over and that he could no longer have anything to do with his wife.

Although he verbally downplayed feeling any guilt in his decision, he nevertheless suffered from and sought treatment for chronic sleeplessness, featuring early morning waking with erethism and revulsion for women. Dosing with Raphanus eliminated the revulsion and brought out a debilitated emotional sensitivity that subsequently responded well to further treatment with two other remedies, Kali phosphoricum and Cyclamen.

SIGHT DIMENSION ILLNESS: DYSMENNORHEA

In TCM and homeopathy, the etiology of a symptom in humans is nonlocal and complex, and its consequences may be similarly nonlocal and complex. For example, if an emotional trauma blurs or destroys one's ability to think logically, and hysteria results, the liver function can become impaired; a damaged liver, in turn, promotes a chaotic movement of the blood.

SIGHT DIMENSION ILLNESS: DYSMENNORHEA
HOMEOPATHIC REMEDIES

Cimicifuga racemosa

Made from the black cohosh plant, Cimicifuga racemosa is a remedy primarily of use to women suffering from dysmennorhea, or disordered menstrual function. Women benefiting from Cimicifuga suffer from any number of gynecological ailments including radiating abdominal pain, profuse and clotted discharges, ovarian neuralgia, bearing-down sensations, miscarriage, uterine prolapse, and a complete loss of menstrual periods. Cimicifuga is also useful during menopause when dwindling menstrual blood liberates a surplus of energy that may exacerbate any hysterical symptoms. A TCM diagnosis of a woman requiring this remedy will likely conclude that there is a disordering of Liver Qi, as a result of which the blood reacts chaotically.

Cimicifuga's mental state exhibits two characteristic delusions. The first is that of having a black cloud of misery and dejection hanging directly over one's head. The second is a general tightness akin to the experience of being encased in wires. Both features, namely, hovering oppression and general tension, find physical expression in muscular soreness and numerous pressing and throbbing pains, particularly of the eyes, neck, head, and the abdomen in relation to menses.

These symptoms appear to be a lack of grounding that expresses itself as loquacity, attention deficit disorder, and exaggeration in speech At the same time, the patient exhibits a proclivity for writing, painting, or theatrical performance. Also in evidence are variable symptoms, ranging from chorea triggered by excitement, to unease and nervousness, fear of insanity, and unwarranted suspicion. Cimicifuga is a also major remedy for sleeplessness during pregnancy or following the nursing of a child.

The clue to Cimicifuga's radical disjunct comes from the remedy's encaged feeling: an oppressive sense of being bound to family members or close relations simultaneously invites a desire to be free from them.

Sepia

As its name implies, Sepia is made from the ink of a sea creature, the cuttlefish. Ink's color, black, absorbs light, a quality that metaphorically, but also literally, accounts for Sepia's remedy picture, that is, a swallowing up of hope, of the light of life. Like ink spilled on and blotting out portions of an important document, Sepia erodes clearly held distinctions critical to a healthy Liver function. The Sepia remedy state describes stagnation resulting from the effects of disappointment that is itself rooted in a blurring of distinction, such as when a depressed woman laments, "Even though he cheats on me, he still loves me."

On the physical plane, dysmenorrhea that is treatable with Sepia results from a profound stagnation that expresses itself in menstrual irregularity: the period may be too late and scanty, too early and profuse, or absent.

TCM teaches that the Spleen is responsible for bolstering the organs and holding them in their rightful place; this function is deranged in the Sepia state.

Commonly experienced within Sepia is a bearing-down sensation, as if everything inside is escaping from the vulva, and symptoms of uterine prolapse.

Although not exclusively so, Sepia is largely a woman's remedy. Individuals having an affinity for its state are, to invoke the famous Aretha Franklin song, "natural women." They like to dance, enjoy nature, are animated, affectionate, and invested in the idea that life progresses in a naturally forward-moving direction. If disappointment interrupts their life's path, symptoms of resentfulness, sarcasm, tearfulness, fatigue, and emotional indifference to a spouse or a child appear, all of which serve as a bitter commentary on the natural state.

Other symptoms further illuminate the underlying problem. A person needing Sepia is likely to experience nausea, acid reflux, or lack of appetite after taking only a few bites of food. Eruptions of the skin occur whose healing crusts prematurely flake off, thus causing the skin to heal twice. This symptom mirrors Sepia's sarcastic state of mind: "Sure, I'll make a half-hearted effort to heal, but that is the best I can manage."

A Sepia woman generally is subject to flushes of heat and faintness, symptoms by now understandable as consequences of the stagnation of Liver Qi. She also exhibits a tendency to misspeak, a characteristic that expresses confusion possibly arising from an unsatisfactory transition through one or another of life's developmental milestones. Further, troublesome experiences during puberty, early sexual events, marriage, childbirth, or menopause may increase resentment with each state she must say goodbye to—be it childhood innocence, puberty, loss of virginity, childlessness, or maternity—and may introduce confusion and uncertainty into her readiness to enter a succeeding developmental state.

Sepia's radical disjunct may be described as "a natural state of hopefulness invites its opposite, a bitter realization that hope itself is toxic." In the event that psychotherapy fails to cleanse hopefulness of its toxicity, it is fortunate that Sepia is available to help restore hopefulness to its natural state.

SIGHT DIMENSION ILLNESS: CHRONIC INFECTION

In homeopathy, numerous reasons may be found to account for a pattern of chronic infection. Some of these infections may be considered miasmatic, as, for example, when repeated exposure to the *Staphylococcinum* bacillus appears to have consolidated within hearing. In TCM, the clinical picture of chronic infection is that of an excess in the Water Phase, manifesting with Kidney symptoms such as a tendency to have chronic dysentery, abscesses, and muco-purulent discharges. Water's excess, in turn, overcontrols and impedes Fire, causing susceptibility to endocarditis, frequent weeping, and aggravation from consolation. The more typically seen constellation of symptoms of chronic infection includes frequent colds, flu, sore throat, ear and sinus infections, allergies, chemical sensitivities, general dryness, and fatigue.

Here we will focus on two TCM patterns, a deficiency of Liver blood and Liver Yin, both of which pertain to chronic infection and illuminate the dimension of sight. Before being released into general circulation, and to meet the demands of the menstrual cycle, the blood undergoes purification by the Liver in which it is stored; but this function of purification can be impaired by an emotional trauma causing stagnation. In addition to performing its function while under this emotional duress and constricted energy, the Liver's ability to purify the blood can be further compromised by a poor diet, environmental pollutants, and less than optimal vitality of Kidney Yin. A deficiency of Liver blood can lend itself to chronic infection appearing in the context of anemia, a tendency towards spasms of the muscles or tendons, numerous skin conditions, numbness, impairment of vision, and paleness of the face or of the fingernail beds.

A deficiency of Liver Yin closely resembles, and can be thought of as extending, the pathology of a deficiency of Liver blood. The burden of blood purification also falls on Kidney Yin, which is responsible for supplying fluid adequate enough to maintain the blood in good health. When Kidney Yin is not entirely up to the task, symptoms of deficiency Heat, as well as dryness, especially of the eyes, irritability, and restlessness, appear. The description of these two major patterns of Liver pathology strongly suggests that upgrading lifestyle, diet, and the environment can go a long way towards bolstering either the blood or Yin of the Liver.

SIGHT DIMENSION ILLNESS: CHRONIC INFECTION
HOMEOPATHIC REMEDY

Silica

Silica is a homeopathic remedy that manifests a striking relationship to light, as well as to deficiencies of Liver Blood and Liver Yin. The nonmetallic element silicon, although it makes up more than one-fourth of the earth's crust, does not occur freely in nature. As silica, it appears in the quartz crystal, sandstone, or sand,

and as silicate in feldspar, mica, asbestos, and thousands of other compounds. In 1921, the piezoelectric property of quartz, namely its ability to generate an electrical charge, was discovered. Quartz is also pyroelectric, meaning that it will generate a charge when heated or rubbed. Its use in stabilizing the frequency of radio transmissions and its application within transistors has given quartz a key role in communications technology. In view of these properties, it might be said of quartz that within nature, the mineral holds a relationship to electricity parallel with that which the Liver holds within the body in relation to Qi.

Historically, in shamanistic cultures, quartz was exploited for its purported magical properties to elevate spiritual vision, to allow communication with the dead, and to enhance the power of prayer—as expressed in TCM, the ability to ease entry to the Hun, the Ethereal Soul housed within the Liver. In numerous cultures, quartz has been valued for its possession of medical properties to enhance fertility and eliminate thirst or edema; these concepts specifically support and enhance the function of the Kidney and therefore also of Liver Yin. The same can be said for the role of silicon in fostering grain crops, where it has been found to promote the strength of stalks and to bolster a plant's resistance to fungus, insect infestation, and loss of water.

Silica is, of course, the most important component of glassware, a material whose keynote properties, namely transparency to light and brittleness, find parallels within an individual constitutionally in need of this remedy. Such a person is terribly self-conscious; he feels that others see right through him as if he were, in fact, transparent. He is also brittle in the sense of being oversensitive to criticism, noise, and light.

The mental and emotional presentation of this remedy also includes other striking features: The Silica individual is likely to be obsessed with small, pointed objects such as pins; his hypersensitivity impairs his confidence and can cause severe performance anxiety; he is frequently detail-conscious and unable to view the big picture. This last psychological feature reflects silica's molecular structure, notable for a tightness of bonding between individual molecules. Overall, however, silica has a surprisingly amorphous structure, more characteristic of a liquid than of a crystalline substance. The Silica individual's tendency to remain rutted in emotional dependency, stubbornness, and indecision also suggests that light has penetrated to his core, only to be internally refracted and denied egress.

The Silica state either emerges from or reflects a susceptibility to think too much or to suffer from the strain of mental activity or malnourishment. It is a major remedy for infants who, in a self-thwarting manner, poorly tolerate their mother's milk. Even when used as an acute remedy, Silica is renowned for its ability to undo the thwarting of self, and to initiate pushing out and pushing through. Thus, it is the remedy of choice for promoting detoxification by inducing perspiration, suppuration by bringing boils and furuncles to a head, or pushing a splinter to the skin's surface.

The Silica remedy state reveals that, whether from exhaustion, inferior nutrition, or inborn hypersensitivity, excessive thought can thwart creativity. Liver Qi thus becomes gnarled and more likely to promote its own entanglement than to serve creative effort. Alternately mild and severely obstinate, the Silica personality is well-defined by Schopenhauer's observation that obstinacy is the result of the will forcing itself over the intellect. Thus we are led to the remedy's radical disjunct: a determination to answer every question invites an unwillingness to answer even a single question.

The picture of a well-compensated Silica individual appears rather normal; rather than being incapacitated by hypersensitivity or mental overactivity, a leading Silica man enlists his self-consciousness as a means to outstrip his peers. For a hilarious and vivid picture of such a Silica personality one might read *My Years with Ross*[12] in which the author, James Thurber, recounts his experience at the famed *New Yorker* magazine during the editorship of its eccentric yet brilliant founder, Harold Ross, a fully realized Silica individual.

Silica and Its Complement Pulsatilla

Silica is a complement and chronic manifestation of Pulsatilla, another very different homeopathic remedy. When viewed in the context of the metabolism, Pulsatilla is a remedy at whose crux is a feeling of being forsaken. Individuals in need of Pulsatilla are readily tearful and sympathetic to abandonment issues within themselves and others, and their emotions are not at all inwardly thwarted, as we have seen in the Silica individual. Pulsatilla presents instead a highly hormonal remedy state featuring poorly controlled movement of the blood and bodily fluids. Pulsatilla manifests Liver Wind because its symptoms fluctuate significantly; this again contrasts with Silica, which lacks fluctuations. In the surprising conjunction of the Silica and Pulsatilla states often seen in homeopathic clinical practice, we find an example of the pendulum-shift phenomenon described in Chapter 2. In this metaphor, a remedy—in this case, Silica—represents the far point of a pendulum's arc in one direction while a well-indicated second remedy—here, Pulsatilla—prompts the pendulum's weight to swing in the opposite direction.

THE SIGHT DIMENSION: PERSONAL THERAPEUTIC PRACTICES AND MASTERS OF EXPRESSION

In addition to the suggested uses of homeopathy and biomedicine in this chapter, several therapeutic practices can help promote health within the sense dimension of sight. **Table 1** lists a number of these practices.

Throughout history, a number of masters have strongly expressed either the positive or negative poles of the sense dimension of sight. **Table 2** lists several of these masters who exemplified one or the other side of the creativity-chaos axis, the core issue of the dimension of sight.

Table 1. Sight Dimension: Health-promoting Practices

Clearly, cleanly attend to detail	See the big picture
Convert anger into creative action	Adopt simplicity, avoid clutter
Nurture the mother of sight, *Hearing*: "Consolidate your resources"	Think like a world citizen
Consolidate your resources	Foster flow in all situations

Table 2. Examples of Masters of the Sense Dimension of Sight

NEGATIVE POLE: CHAOS	POSITIVE POLE: CREATIVITY
Playwright John Osborne *(Look Back in Anger)*	Visionaries, seminal thinkers: William James
Totalitarian dictators: Hitler, Stalin	Great artists, musicians, writers, mathematicians: Einstein, Leonardo
Religious fanatics	Masters of sparseness and simplicity: Shaker artisans

CHAPTER EIGHT

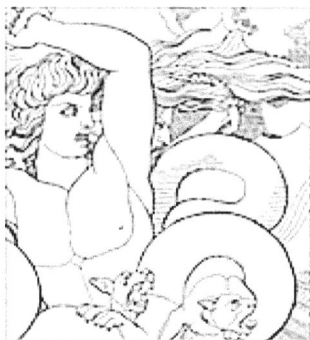

Encountering Scylla: Consciousness and Cancer

Before the gates there sat
On either side a formidable Shape.
The one seemed a woman to the waist, and fair,
But ended foul in many a scaly fold,
Voluminous and vast—a serpent armed
With mortal sting. About her middle round
A cry of Hell-hounds never-ceasing barked
With wide Cerberean mouths full loud, and rung
A hideous peal; yet, when they list, would creep,
If aught disturbed their noise, into her womb,
And kennel there; yet there still barked and howled
Within unseen. Far less abhorred than these
Vexed Scylla, bathing in the sea that parts
Calabria from the hoarse Trinacrian shore;

—*John Milton, Paradise Lost, Book II*

THE CULTURE OF CANCER

E lements of cancer, and of all other illnesses, are embedded in cultures through-out the world. Cultural symbols and stories represent outward projections of the experience of illness, whether these projections are conscious or subconscious, psychological or biological. Just as bodily symptoms might be decoded to under-stand psychological problems, so cultural symbols and practices might be decoded to recover an understanding of health and illness.

How we understand and relate to cancer influences our health and, poten-tially, our healing from cancer. Because the causes of cancer can be found in sys-tems larger and smaller than those of one person, total control of the illness is not possible. But the individual, as the host to a cancer, plays an active role: conscious-ness, whether cultural, individual, cellular, or molecular, influences the biological experience of resisting, succumbing to, or recovering from illness.

THE MYTH OF SCYLLA

I n the *Odyssey*, the magnificent ancient Greek epic by Homer, Ulysses was sail-ing home to his wife Penelope, when his ship had to pass through the nar-row Strait of Messina which was guarded by two terrifying monsters, Scylla and Charybdis, entrenched on either side of the strait. Scylla was described as once having been a beautiful nymph who was poisoned in her bath by jealous Circe and transformed into a hideous monster with twelve feet and six heads, each with three rows of teeth. Below the waist, her body was made up of horrible monsters, like dogs, who barked unceasingly. In this state she was destined to live forever in unending misery and loathing, unable to move, and destroying everything that came within her reach.

In this chapter, we will reach deeply into the myth of Scylla and define the commonality between her story and that of cancerous tumor growth. Just as once innocent Scylla was transformed by poison into a gruesome monster, so once innocent cells may become malignant through damage from macro-cosmic and microcosmic exposures. Scylla's voraciousness reflects the relent-lessly invasive and devouring hunger of cancer. To the extent that there are no limits on how many times cancer cells are able to divide, they share another of Scylla's traits—immortality. Similarly, Scylla's isolation and self-loathing are manifested in cancer cells. To use Robert Weinberg's[1] term, a "renegade" cancer cell alienates itself from its own community, thereby instigating a bodily outcry and a witch hunt against itself. Scylla's aberrant anatomy correlates with cancer's breakdown of normal order and the chaotic management of cell replacement. Tumors known as teratomata (Greek for "monster tumor") consist of tissues well-enough differentiated to contain hair and teeth. They may be either malignant or benign. Scylla is a teratomata sprung to life and preserved in myth. Prescient echoes from multiple levels of consciousness and experience are held in the cultural vessel that is the myth of Scylla.

THE MYTH OF SATAN

By objectifying our fears, myths like that of Scylla serve to alleviate our helplessness and enhance our sense of control. The myth of Satan performs a similar function. In the major world religions, Satan is depicted as a fallen angel, formerly favored by God; this myth of Satan can be viewed allegorically as the cultural and biological equivalent of cancer willfully seeking freedom from, and chaotically ruling, our bodies. Like Satan, cancer makes a hell that destroys itself.[2]

Satan's story is told with dramatic effect in John Milton's epic poem, *Paradise Lost*. It is to this that we turn in interpreting the nature of Satan as it typifies cancer. First we refer to Satan's character described in *Paradise Lost*, then give our commentary as a biological description of cancer preserved in the myth of Satan, "the father of lies."[3]

Paradise Lost, Book I

Hail, horrors! hail,
Infernal world! and thou, profoundest Hell,
Receive thy new possessor--one who brings
A mind not to be changed by place or time.
The mind is its own place, and in itself
Can make a Heaven of Hell, a Hell of Heaven.
What matter where, if I be still the same,
And what I should be, all but less than he
Whom thunder hath made greater? Here at least
We shall be free;

Commentary

*A normal cell must convert to a cancerous state by undergoing some-
thing akin to a seduction. Like a Faustian bargain, in exchange for
being granted immortality—the ability to reproduce without limitations—the cell pledges itself to a tumor colony, each cell of which is
possessed of a similar delusion: a belief that the tumor's existence is
separate and independent from the existence of its host.*

Paradise Lost, Book I

. . . .but under brows
Of dauntless courage, and considerate pride
Waiting revenge. Cruel his eye, but cast
Signs of remorse and passion, to behold
The fellows of his crime, the followers rather
(Far other once beheld in bliss), condemned
For ever now to have their lot in pain--
Millions of Spirits for his fault amerced
Of Heaven, and from eternal splendours flung
For his revolt--yet faithful how they stood,
Their glory withered;

Commentary

*Cancer cells are single-minded zealots, martyrs willing to sacrifice
themselves on behalf of the tumor colony's voracious demands.*

Paradise Lost, Book I

. . . . ever to do ill our sole delight,
As being the contrary to his high will
Whom we resist. If then his providence
Out of our evil seek to bring forth good,
Our labour must be to pervert that end,
And out of good still to find means of evil;

*   *   *

Here we may reign secure; and, in my choice,
To reign is worth ambition, though in Hell:
Better to reign in Hell than serve in Heaven.

Commentary

Cancer cells are inspired to metastasize. Far-flung missions are embarked on whose goal is to colonize tissue entirely foreign to that of the cancer cell's original composition.

CANCER CELL SEDUCTION

If, allegorically, the cancer cell represents a seduction by the teachings of a false prophet, how and where might this seductive pressure arise? One implicated culprit is the free radical molecule.

A free radical is any atom or molecule possessing a single, unpaired electron in its outer shell. Free radicals are a product of oxidative stress associated with cellular aging.

From the vantage point of an oxidative stress "lifestyle," free radicals are, metaphorically, like adolescents who neglect their hydration and expose themselves to environmental contaminants while indulging irresponsibly in smoking, alcohol, and consuming high amounts of unhealthy fats and empty calories.

From the vantage point of their need to achieve stability, most biologically relevant free radicals behave again like unsatisfied adolescents desperately pirating an electron away from their most proximal stable molecule. A vampire-like chain reaction then results whereby the attacked molecule, losing its electron, becomes itself a free radical. The chain reaction's cascade disrupts the living cell to which the molecule belongs. The aggregate effect of this "adolescent" onslaught on the cells and their DNA is a destabilizing pressure that may seduce a cell into a cancerous society.

According to the principle, "As within, so without," the oxidative stress of these "adolescent" free radicals is remarkably metaphorically parallel to Wilhelm Reich's account of the mass psychology of fascism. There Reich posits a dynamic in which adolescents exposed to a sexually repressed ideology become sadistic, group-encased, and vulnerable to the teachings of a paternalistic authority.[4]

CAUSES AND RISK FACTORS OF CANCER

There are more than 100 types of cancer, according to the U.S. National Cancer Institute and the National Institute of Environmental Health Sciences booklet, *Cancer and the Environment: What You Need to Know, What You Can Do*, published in 2003.[5] Further, the *Report on Carcinogens, Eleventh Edition*, released January 31, 2005, by scientists at the National Toxicology Program (NTP) in Research Triangle Park, North Carolina, identified 246 agents which either are known to be human carcinogens or reasonably anticipated to be human carcinogens, and to which a significant number of persons in the United States are exposed.[6] The National Cancer Institute's booklet on *Cancer and the Environment* lists about 50 of these agents that are currently of greatest public interest. The range is enormous and includes tobacco; diet/weight/physical inactivity; alcoholic drinks; ultraviolet radiation; viruses and bacteria; ionizing radiation; pesticides; medical drugs; solvents; fibers, fine particles, and dust; dioxins; polycyclic aromatic hydrocarbons (PAHs); metals; diesel exhaust particles; toxins from fungi; vinyl chloride; and benzidine.[5] The list reads like an alarming *Materia Medica* of modern life, the macrocosmic equivalent of microcosmic toxic stress within the individual.

Cancer in Microcosmic Context: The World of Viruses and Genes

Viruses and their subclasses compose a group of organisms that can be designated as ambiguously lifelike. The blurry boundary that distinguishes a cell from a virus indicates the extent to which cellular and viral evolution are interwoven. The parasitism of a virus issues directly from its incompleteness. Incapable of independent metabolism, viruses are entirely dependent on their ability to gain entry to a host.

When not active and in a host, a virus remains locked in an inert state. The host is exploited for the sake of viral self-replication. Because it flourishes only so long as its host remains alive, the virus holds a particularly strong interest in cellular immortality. Viruses express the enzyme telomerase, which prevents shortening of chromosomal endings known as telomeres. This delays senescence, or cellular aging.

Although the ability to produce telomerase is encoded within each and every cell, the greater good of the organism demands that except where necessary—that is, in stem cells operating within the germ line—genetic expression of telomerase is suppressed. The inherent self-renewal of stem cells, and their ability to morph into any sort of tissue, has led to new concepts implicating "cancer stem cells" in malignancy. A growing consensus within the oncology research community now attributes cancer's development and resistance to even aggressive chemotherapy to a relatively small number of stem cell split-offs known as progenitor cells. Some studies even suggest that cancer stem cells may be derived from normal stem cells. Research indicates that progenitor or normal stem cells mutated into cancer stem cells may generate a primary tumor, resist chemotherapy and become refractory, or metastasize to distal sites. Although mutated stem cells are now considered to be significant in the development of cancer, they are few in number, relatively quiescent compared to other cancer cells, and difficult to target.[7,8]

An estimated 15% to 20% of human cancers worldwide, in 2002, were attributable to viral infections.[9] Certain viruses increase a person's risk for, or are considered to cause, cancer. For example, human papilloma virus (HPV) infection is the main cause of cervical cancer and may be a risk factor for other cancers, while chronic hepatitis B and hepatitis C infections can lead to liver cancer. The human T-cell leukemia/lymphoma virus (HTLV-1) is associated with increased risk of lymphoma and leukemia, while the Epstein-Barr virus (EBV) may predispose to lymphoma.[10]

Before associating viruses only with disease, we should remember where they occur in the natural order. Viral ability to consolidate synchrony, meaning to encode adaptive strategies for heritable purposes, translates into reproductive expertise indispensable to higher evolution. It is thus not surprising that approximately eight percent or 100,000 segments of human DNA are remarkably similar to retroviruses (a viral class that includes HIV).[11]

Do we have incorporated viral material in our genome? The authors of a research paper, published in *PLoS Pathogens*, in July 2010,[12] reported that they have uncovered about 80 high-confidence examples of genomic DNA sequences in 19 vertebrate species, including humans and other mammals, which "as long ago as 40 million years. . . acquired sequences related to the genes of certain of these RNA viruses. Surprisingly, almost all of the nearly 80 integrations identified are related to only two viral families, the Ebola/Marburgviruses and Bornaviruses, which are deadly pathogens that cause lethal hemorrhagic fevers and neurological disease, respectively."[12] The authors go on to suggest that the expression and conservation of these sequences may have given an advantage to the vertebrates by providing resistance to the diseases caused by the viruses, while, at the same time, they allowed the viruses to persist and to be transmitted. Could this be a win-win relationship over millions of years?

Although viruses succeed in reproducing themselves, one viral sub-class, the episomes, can reproduce only when their hosts do so. An episome is a mere sliver of self-replicating genetic material whose transfer to a bacterial host can become essential to a bacteria's well-being and ability to reproduce. As such, it is the episome that ushers bacteria into an early experience of synchrony. Along with certain retroviruses, episomes belong to the class of transposons, or transposable genetic elements. Transposons can become integrated at numerous sites in the genome and have played an important role in evolutionary development.

One can only stand in awe of the synchronic and transcendent genome, the human organism's vast blueprint replete with incredible safeguards that effectively shield the genome from harm. The DNA molecules appear structured to guard the genome. Not only are their bases turned inwards so as to avoid direct attack by chemical mutagens, but they are resistant to cleavage from alkaline ions arising within cytoplasm.

DNA's robustness nevertheless is vulnerable to subversion. The exploitable weaknesses are cell growth and cell division. Each time a cell undergoes replication its entire genome must be recopied. When a copying error occurs within a sequence of DNA prior to cell division, one of the daughter cells receives a mutated and potentially cancerous version. Imagine, if in the final line of a novel, a key word contains a single incorrect letter: Instead of "You are dear to me," it reads, "You are dead to me." The meaning of the entire book changes. Similarly, the consequences of a tiny transcription error can radically alter the function of a lineage of cells.

CANCERS AND THE SENSE DIMENSIONS

We may see ourselves as victims of our genes, as victims of carcinogenic viruses, as victims of cultural, economic, and environmental conditions—all beyond our control—that contribute to cancer. In our novel model presented here, however, we relate cancers to disturbances of the sense dimensions. Recognizing and addressing those disturbances is one avenue for consciousness to influence healing. Bear in mind that healing at the level of the human spirit is a worthy gift in and of itself, freely available to everyone. Healing of the spirit does not necessarily reverse disease at the level of tissues and organs (although sometimes the bodily level of healing also occurs). Healing the spirit suggests a shift in perspective from passive victim (or hardened foe) to actively receptive partner in one's internal and external states.

In my practice I find that cancer cases reveal a remarkable feature: Instead of erupting in a crisis, the cancer rather influences each of the sense dimensions, expressing a perverse version of the sense dimension's core issue. Although an increasing number of homeopathic remedies have been found to be useful in treating cancer, for our purposes here, we will consider morbidity in each of the sense dimensions through the materia medica of perhaps the most commonly used cancer remedy, Carcinosin, a nosode derived from breast carcinoma tissue.[13]

Morbid Touch

In the sense dimension of touch, the core issue is the tension between synchrony and isolation. Normal cells unselfishly serve the synchrony of a greater good related to the needs of the surrounding community of tissue. With corruption into a cancer cell, the cell degrades into isolation. Consequently, at cellular and psychological levels, the core tension between isolation and synchrony is increased.

The Carcinosin remedy state depicts an experience of preternatural responsibility at an early age, leading to an excessively sympathetic adult. How are this sympathy, the isolated cancer cell, and the isolation a cancer patient feels related? If, for example, a child is placed in the role of caretaker for an adult, this too-early burden plants a delusion in the person that she must do it all alone, must sacrifice her own needs for those of others, perhaps to the extent of becoming a martyr. A sense of isolation is eventually created that supplants the initial sympathetic tendency. Thus, isolation is an inversion of sympathetic nurturing; and an excess of sympathy can, like virulent cancer cells, fuel a delusion that life can be everlasting, a delusion that is both debilitating and self-destructive.

Morbid Taste

In the sense dimension of taste, in which the core issue is the tension between challenge and anxiety, a rapidly growing tumor's aggressiveness and hedonistic appropriation of resources may be considered bacterial consciousness run amok; it is mirrored by a wild exaggeration of taste's hunger for challenge, its positive pole. An individual immersed in the Carcinosin remedy state can manifest a version of this exaggeration, becoming as ambitious and workaholic as a tumor cell, and taking on more than he can handle. On the other side of taste's core axis—the negative pole, anxiety—an individual may be a perfectionist and overly fastidious.

Morbid Smell

The core tension in the sense dimension of smell is between centeredness and disorientation. A component of metastatic cancer, the attraction away from its place of origin to distant locales, represents a perversion of the smell dimension's positive pole, centeredness.

An individual needing Carcinosin is romantic, keen on dancing, and drawn to foreign travel. On the physical plane, Carcinosin manifests a tendency to asthma and bronchitis with regard to the lungs, and cafe-au-lait pigmentation and numerous moles with regard to the skin. Because the cancerous tissue from which Carcinosin nosode is made is taken from the breast—a part of the body governed by the dimension of smell—romance is associated with lung ailments within this remedy (an association exquisitely epitomized in the Thomas Mann novel, *The Magic Mountain*).

Extraordinarily, smell-dimension theory in its negative pole, disorientation, is in perfect concert with biological phenomena: genetic pathology in the form of a cataclysmic breakdown in coding, known as a frameshift mutation, manifests utter disorientation, a disorientation that may eventually be displayed in advanced cancer.

Morbid Hearing

The core issue in the sense dimension of hearing is the tension between consolidation and entropy. A genetic predisposition to one or more cancers exhibits a perverse expression of consolidation. Familial retinoblastoma, for example, is imprinted upon and consolidated within the Kidney Yang. Genetically, a heritable mutation of a gene on the thirteenth human chromosome creates a susceptibility to the deactivation of a tumor suppressor, which, in turn, allows tumors to grow in the retina and other locales. As the principal remedy relevant to the cancer miasm, Carcinosin is applicable to cancers that have been imprinted and consolidated within the germ line.

Morbid Sight

In the sense dimension of sight, where the core tension is between creativity and chaos, cancer cells exhibit a perverse creativity in forming novel mutant combinations. Here, tumor growth is an exaggeration of the negative pole of chaos, demonstrated by the juxtaposition of incompatible tissues. In this dimension, symptoms related to Carcinosin include twitching of the eyes or limbs, an emotional sensitivity, and a will to be productive.

Partnering With the Genome

Is it possible for us to assist the genome in maintaining its integrity? So long as optimal health is defined within the sense dimensions in terms of the positive poles of synchrony, challenge, centeredness, consolidation, and creativity, the answer might well be yes. If there are problematic issues within the sense dimensions, well-targeted correctives to an individual's consciousness within the sense dimensions might lead to a reversal of chronic illness, including cancer.

LESSONS LEARNED FROM CANCER AWARENESS

Despite our individual uniqueness, we become cognizant, through experience of the positive poles of the sense dimensions, that each of us is also a cellular component of a vastly larger organism—perhaps as large as the universe—in which each cellular unit is maintained by being in creative synchrony with all other units. Cells, and all beings, from viruses to humans, are born, fulfill their life's purpose, and die. Cancer has shown us that death itself appears to be a vital function of this universal rhythm of existence. Perhaps were living beings not to die, they might, like cancer cells, become isolated, disoriented, uncontrollably chaotic, and ultimately destructive of the life host itself. In the universal view, every state of existence, whether it be viral, microbial, or human, manifests its purposefulness through creativity and utility. TCM teaches that the lessons learned are stored after death within the Kidney Yang; and thus, the vital energies never die.

CHAPTER NINE

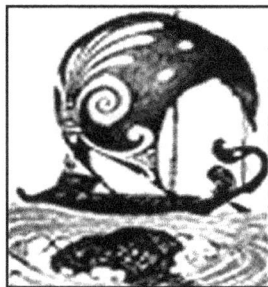

Encountering Charybdis: The Chronic Illness Vortex

> And more endangered than when Argo passed
> Through Bosporus betwixt the justling rocks,
> Or when Ulysses on the larboard shunned
> Charybdis, and by th' other whirlpool steered.
>
> —*John Milton, Paradise Lost, Book II*

SENSITIVITY AND SUSCEPTIBILITY

The specific quality of an individual's sensitivity is a vital source of information in diagnosing chronic illness; a shift in a person's sensitivity to a substance or experience, whether it be for better or for worse, is a momentous event. A sensitivity imbalance can occur when either overexposure or underexposure to a substance or experience causes a previously neutral sensitivity to these substances and events to split into hypersensitive and hyposensitive components that can cause powerful responses. Independent of any kind of treatment, an individual's sensitivity and his or her ability to heal are inseparable.

Our sensitivities are not entirely inborn. Sensitivity, like that to the nuances of music, to a great painting, or to the suffering of others, can be cultivated. To a certain extent, our sensitivity to infection from germs or to the dangers of flying can also be modified. In fact, unless the capability to influence sensitivity exists, knowledge has little value with regard to healing. Susceptibility to illness may be rooted in the tenor of our thoughts and in the quality of our choices, both physical and mental.

THE MYTH OF CHARYBDIS

In the *Odyssey*, as Ulysses's ship passed through the narrow Strait of Messina, the enormous tidal whirlpool of the sea monster-goddess Charybdis swirled on one side of the strait opposite the equally dangerous monster Scylla. In one ancient story describing the origin of Charybdis, she was a daughter of Pontos, the divine sea-god, and Gaia, the earth-goddess. Charybdis had so angered Zeus that he turned her into a monster compelled forever to suck water in and expel it out three times a day, drawing men down into the spiral whirlpool to their deaths. Charybdis symbolizes the cyclical, vortex nature of chronic illness.

TCM THEORY: THE ENERGY CYCLES

TCM weaves almost inexhaustibly comprehensive and precise depictions of the multiple patterns and interactions that occur in healthy and dynamic cycles of life and those that occur in illness and stagnation cycles. This chapter will demonstrate these cycles in detail, beginning with TCM's Five-Phases pentagram (see **Figure 1**) as first described in Chapter Two, "Beyond Biomedicine," and will move on from there to a theoretically more advanced synthesis of the Phases in their cyclical modes. As in previous chapters, organs, phases, states, and energies that pertain descriptively to TCM will be shown capitalized.

TCM's Five-Phases framework portrays several different energetic relationships between the Phases and their associated organs. The first set of relationships, known as the Generating Cycle, shows the links between phases, organs, seasons, life-stages, and sense dimensions.

Figure 2 depicts the healthy and dynamic pattern of energetic nourishment that is transferred from one Phase and its associated organs to the next, directly succeeding Phase. Each Phase provides the impetus for its succeeding Phase.

Similarly, the resolution or positive negotiation of a sense-dimension core issue provides the impetus to encounter the sense-dimension issue of the next Phase.

Figure 1. Five-Phases Pentagram

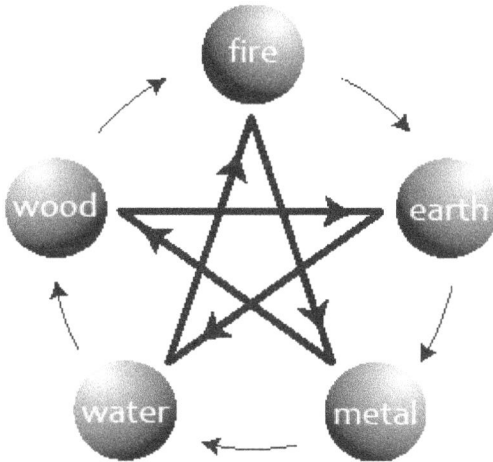

Figure 2. The Generating Cycle

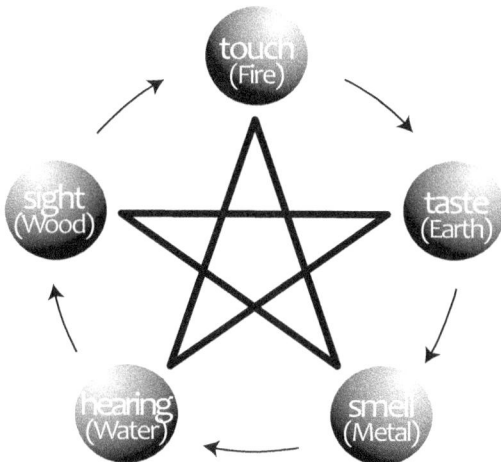

SMOOTH SAILING:
THE HEALTHY GENERATING CYCLE

The Generating Cycle provides a template of a person's normal growth function. Homeopathic theory lacks the taxonomy to create templates for normalcy; so here TCM theory makes an invaluable contribution. Starting with Fire and proceeding to each succeeding Phase, following are the Generating Cycle Phases and relationships, with a description of variables involved in each Phase.

Fire Phase

Fire	Promotes	Earth
(Heart, Touch, Synchrony)	⇒	**(Spleen, Taste, Challenge)**

The Heart is the master organ of Fire, the embodied and pulsing source of synchrony. In TCM, the Heart is conceived of as master of the blood, and also as the residence of the mind. Because of this dual role, it would be more correct to refer to this organ as the Heart/Mind. The blood and Qi of the Heart directly nourish the Spleen. More pointedly, the Fire of the Heart contributes to the heat needed for digestion.

The Heart is associated with Summer, as the full force of the sun corresponds with the Fire Phase. The generation of Earth by Fire is exemplified by the action of Fire which leaves dusty, earth-like ash as its residue. With respect to the life stages, the Heart is associated with childhood. This is a time of rapid growth and development, both biologically and socially. Without synchrony, the body could not achieve orderly growth, and the individual could not become a social being.

As we proceed from the sense dimension of touch, with which the Heart and synchrony are connected, to the next sense dimension of taste, in which the Spleen and challenge are represented, the question is "How does synchrony contribute to the succeeding sense dimension issue of challenge?"

Synchrony is initially experienced through loving attachments with parents. The security of being loved and accepted provides the impetus for moving out into the world and seeking its challenges.

Earth Phase

Earth	Promotes	Metal
(Spleen, Taste, Challenge)	⇛	(Lungs, Smell, Centeredness)

The Spleen and its associated organ of Earth, the Stomach, make nutrients available through the breakdown and digestion of food and drink. The Spleen is responsible for transporting, distributing, and transforming nutrients, and for promoting fluid metabolism. It also governs the blood, keeping blood in its correct course. It is also thought to hold organs in their proper places, and to rule over the condition of the muscles. The Spleen is said to nourish the Lungs by its upward transportation of food essence.

The Spleen is associated with Long Summer, or late Summer. Earth's generation of Metal is exemplified by the mining of the earth for metals, as if metals were produced by the action of the earth.

With respect to the life stages, the Spleen corresponds with adolescence. It is the ripening stage of a person's transformation into his or her fully adult capacities. The desire for mastery over taste's core issue of challenge leads the individual forward into the next stage of life.

How does challenge within the sense dimension of taste contribute to the core issue of centeredness within the succeeding sense dimension of smell? The surmounting of challenges establishes a sense of capability, self-esteem, and self-identity. On this foundation centeredness is built.

Metal Phase

Metal	Promotes	Water
(Lungs, Smell, Centeredness)	⇛	(Kidneys, Hearing, Consolidation)

The Lungs oversee respiration and control the Qi of the entire body. Inspired air is filtered and directed downward, which is said to also help distribute food essence throughout the body. The Lungs activate the flow of vital energy, blood, and the body's fluids. Fluids produced by metabolism are also propelled downward into the Kidneys and the Urinary Bladder.

Autumn is the season of the Lungs. The harvest time is tinged with a melancholy sense of the year's decline. The generation of Water by Metal is exemplified by the melting of metal into a liquid state.

The Lungs correspond to the life stages of adulthood through middle age. An individual is at the center of generations in the middle years, raising children and caring for elders. Yet, every midpoint eventually gives way to a turning point.

How does smell's sense dimension issue of centeredness contribute to the succeeding issue of consolidation within the sense dimension of hearing? When centeredness is mastered and is no longer an issue, one can enter into a more relaxed and established state of being in the world. This state is the consolidation within the next stage of life, old age.

Water Phase

Water	**Promotes**	**Wood**
(Kidneys, Hearing, Consolidation)	⇛	**(Liver, Sight, Creativity)**

The Kidneys rule over Water and the bones. They also store Essence (Jing), heritable energy that influences growth, development, and reproduction. Genetic susceptibilities to disease are considered in TCM to be deficiencies of Essence; thus, in TCM, the Kidneys play a foundational role in existence. In addition to their primary Water functions, the Kidneys also have a Fire function which assists the Heart and contributes heat for digestion. Kidney Yin energy is also a balancing input that is essential for the Liver.

Winter is the season of the Kidneys. In the cold of the winter season, energy returns to its core and is held close within so that one can endure the winter. The generation of Wood by Water is exemplified by water's promotion of the growth of trees.

The life stage of old age corresponds to the Kidneys. Toward the end of life, grandparents are drawn to grandchildren, and, relieved of life's burden of work, elders may encounter a second childhood. Old age impels reunion with the next stage in the generating cycle.

Hearing's sense dimension issue of consolidation contributes to the succeeding issue of creativity in the sense dimension of sight. Hearing's consolidated talents and predispositions are transmitted by Essence and stored in the Kidneys. These are the wellsprings of creativity.

From a generational perspective, consolidation is marked by a concern for our legacy; and the guarantors and repositories of our accomplishments are our children. Our consolidated treasures are passed on to our children and expand to the community, where they inspire creativity and new beginnings.

Wood Phase

Wood (Liver, Sight, Creativity)	Promotes ⇒	Fire (Heart, Touch, Synchrony)

The Liver is the storehouse of the blood and the ruler of the tendons and ligaments. In a healthy state, the Liver administers the smooth flow of Qi throughout the body, which facilitates four functions: harmonious emotions, harmonious digestion, harmonious flow of bile, and harmonious menstruation. When the Liver has sufficient blood and can facilitate blood's smooth movement, then the Heart will be nourished with abundant blood.

The season of the Liver is spring, the time of animal birthing and vegetal rebirthing after the dormancy of winter. The generation of Fire by Wood is exemplified by the use of wood as fuel for fire.

Birth is the stage of life that corresponds with the Liver. Birth is a time of vulnerability that impels synchrony with the mother, which later expands to attunement with the wider environment.

What does the dimension of sight's issue of creativity furnish touch dimension's core issue of synchrony? Creativity generates a unifying flow of energy that is sustained through synchrony. Creative energy is vibrant and attractive, bringing people together and producing communities of the like-minded.

MOTHER-CHILD RELATIONSHIPS

In the mutual relationship of the Five Phases, each of the Phases has the property of generating or giving energy to the next Phase. These Phase pairs are known in

TCM as "Mother" and "Child." Each Phase within the Generating Cycle is the Mother to the next succeeding Phase, the Child. For example, within the Generating Cycle, Fire is the Mother of Earth, while Earth is the Child of Fire.

Each Phase also restrains or controls another; the proper amount of feedback and control keeps the Phases functioning smoothly and in balance. Disharmony occurs when the Mother of a Phase is deficient or weak and provides too little for the Child; or the Child is too strong and takes too much from the Mother. If the relationship between Mother and Child of any of the Phases becomes unbalanced, health problems occur.

A guiding principle within TCM is that when a particular Phase is deficient, blocked, or stagnated —a condition that can generate a range of chronic pathologies—the treatment strategy in TCM is to tonify the Mother in the preceding Phase. In this chapter, the terms "tonify" and "sedate," loosely translated from TCM, imply providing different kinds of supplementation or support when tonifying and draining and weakening when sedating. Below we examine treatment strategies in each of the Phases that involve tonifying the Mother.

"If the Child, Earth, is deficient (Taste, Anxiety, Spleen) then ⟶ Tonify the Mother, Fire (Touch, Synchrony, Heart)"

Encountering an excessively anxious patient leads us to diagnose a blockage related to the dimension of taste. The patient may have had a history of either unreasonable parental demands (excessive challenge—the opposite pole from anxiety on the axis of taste's core issue) or overprotectiveness (inadequate challenge). Treatment involves tonifying the Mother, Fire, the Phase preceding that of Earth, by immersing the patient in synchrony, the positive pole of the sense dimension of touch.

The patient should be cloaked in caring until she regains an embracing sense of security. This is best accomplished by gaining heightened support from family and friends. Counseling, spiritual resources, homeopathy, and acupuncture provide additional treatments. If the Mother, Fire, is tonified, the patient becomes energized and prepared to engage with issues on the anxiety-challenge axis. From the perspective of the sense dimension of taste, the therapeutic focus is on resolving the problem of challenge in the patient's life.

"If the Child, Metal, is deficient (Smell, Disorientation, Lungs) then ⟶ *Tonify the Mother, Earth (Taste, Challenge, Spleen)"*

A functionally depressed patient reveals that he is mired in grief, overcome by the loss of a close personal relationship. If he is disoriented with regard to time, stuck in the past, and unable to perceive the dynamism inherent in the current moment, he is diagnosed with a blockage related to the dimension of smell. The patient is treated by tonifying the Mother, Earth, through immersing him in challenge, the positive pole of the Earth Phase; he is advised to become engaged in an enjoyably challenging project. From the perspective of the sense dimensions, the therapeutic focus is on resolving the lack of centeredness, the positive pole of the sense dimension of smell.

"If the Child, Water, is deficient (Hearing, Entropy, Kidneys) then ⟶ *Tonify the Mother, Metal (Smell, Centeredness, Lungs)"*

During an interview with a middle-aged man, he maintains that his life has fallen apart; he reveals that he is in a state of despair. He feels that his career has been pointless, and that, within his family, he is not valued for anything other than his ability to put food on the table. The patient's age and his rudderless condition lead us to diagnose a blockage within the sense dimension of hearing and a descent into entropy, the negative pole of the hearing sense.

The treatment for this patient's condition is to tonify the Mother, Metal, by immersing the patient in centeredness, the positive pole of the sense dimension of smell in the Metal Phase. Healing is effected by teaching him to meditate; the relaxed centeredness of the meditative state prepares him to face the entropy and to focus therapeutically on resolving the issue of consolidation, the positive pole of the sense dimension of hearing.

"If the Child, Wood, is deficient (Sight, Chaos, Liver)
then ⟶
Tonify the Mother, Water (Hearing, Consolidation, Kidneys)"

An interview with a workaholic woman, who complains of headache and fatigue, brings to light an immense reservoir of anger, frustration, and resentment that she harbors toward her coworkers and her husband. Her anger appears to have originated in a long-standing pattern of unresolved conflict with her now aged parents, whom she felt she had never managed to please. Additional chaotic relationships, hidden agendas, and an inability to address her problems directly indicate a diagnosis of a blockage within the dimension of sight.

Treatment here is effected by tonifying the Mother, Water, by vitalizing consolidation, the positive pole of the sense dimension of hearing. The treatment involves the taking stock and reordering of the patient's priorities. She is encouraged to redirect some of her energies from her career to quality time spent with her family; once this consolidation takes place, she is prepared to cope with the core issue of creativity and chaos within the sense of sight and to experience creativity, the positive pole of the sight dimension.

"If the Child, Fire, is deficient (Touch, Isolation, Heart)
then ⟶
Tonify the Mother, Wood (Sight, Creativity, Liver)"

The world of individuals with autism manifests an extreme state of isolation, yet many of those with autism are also savants and possessors of genius-level abilities in the fields of music, art, or mathematics. Autism typically presents blockage within the sense dimension of touch.

The person with autism is treated by tonifying the Mother from the preceding Phase of Wood, and generating creativity, the positive pole of sight. By helping those with autism find, explore, and express their innate creativity, we are helping them build bridges to synchrony, the positive pole of touch, and to fellowship. From the perspective of the sense dimension of touch, the therapeutic focus is on resolving problematic synchrony.

SAILING AGAINST THE TIDE:
THE RETROGRADE GENERATING CYCLE

What happens if energy is transferred in the opposite, retrograde direction on the Generating Cycle—that is, from Child to Mother instead of Mother to Child? This retrograde pattern is sometimes called the Draining Cycle in TCM; its symptoms show up in the clinic particularly when the patient is observed from the perspective of the sense dimensions. **Figure 3** illustrates this Retrograde Generating Cycle of Child to Mother.

Figure 3. The Retrograde Generating Cycle

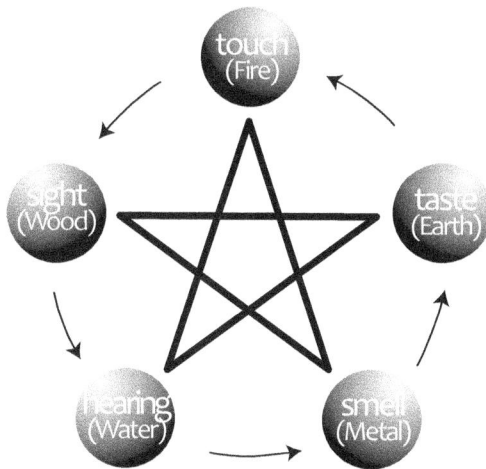

In the Retrograde Generating Cycle, the influence of the negative pole of the sense dimension of the Child overwhelms the Mother, and brings out the negative pole of the sense dimension of the Mother, sending it into crisis. Because the pathology generated by this retrograde cycle is so extreme, no treatment principles are suggested here. On the following pages are descriptions of these retrograde patterns and their pathologies.

"If the Child, Fire (Touch, Isolation, Heart)
overwhelms its Mother, Wood
then →
The Mother, Wood (Sight, Creativity, Liver) falls into crisis,
exposing Chaos"

The psychological profile of this pattern is that of an individual who, following heartbreak or another major loss, degenerates into a state of isolation and the hoarding of keepsakes and mementos, which culminates into living obliviously among piles of papers and garbage or excrement of pets. The physical symptoms following a shock or major loss may include muscular laxness or rigidity, paralysis, stroke, seizures, stupor, or blindness brought on by neurosis.

"If the Child, Wood (Sight, Chaos, Liver)
overwhelms its Mother, Water
then →
The Mother, Water (Hearing, Consolidation, Kidneys) falls into
crisis, exposing Entropy"

This psychological pattern is one of an individual whose protracted anger or intense disappointment has devolved into a profound loss of purpose, and even suicidal inclinations. The bodily symptoms may include degenerative and autoimmune disorders such as scleroderma, lupus, or multiple sclerosis. In this retrograde pattern, when the Liver is Yin deficient and unable to accept Yin from the Kidneys, extreme edema may result.

"If the Child, Water (Hearing, Entropy, Kidneys)
overwhelms its Mother, Metal
then →
The Mother, Metal (Smell, Centeredness, Lungs) falls into
crisis, exposing Disorientation"

In this psychological pattern, an individual believes he has outlived his usefulness. Entropy, appearing as a lost purpose, counteracts centeredness, producing disorientation. Physically, within this pattern, there may be respiratory ailments presenting with Dampness and Phlegm.

"If the Child, Metal (Smell, Disorientation, Lungs) overwhelms its Mother, Earth then —→ The Mother, Earth (Taste, Challenge, Spleen) falls into crisis, exposing Anxiety"

Psychologically, in this pattern, an individual experiences grief that initially produces disorientation and subsequently becomes a state of heightened anxiety, possibly associated with an eating disorder. The extreme picture of this state is that of an Alzheimer's disease patient who stops eating altogether.

"If the Child, Earth (Taste, Anxiety, Spleen) overwhelms its Mother, Fire then —→ The Mother, Fire (Touch, Synchrony, Heart) falls into crisis, exposing Isolation

In this retrograde condition, the individual feels an undercurrent of anxiety, possibly from a sense of shame or guilt, which is sufficient to obliterate synchrony and limit fellowship with others. Physical symptoms may include conversion disorder, heart arrhythmia or palpitations, panic disorder, and a profound sense of personal inadequacy.

In TCM theory, sweet flavor corresponds to the Earth Phase. If sweets are eaten in excess, they may produce a state of nervous anxiety. In the case of a person with diabetes who experiences a diabetic or hypoglycemic shock, nonresponsiveness can replace synchrony.

TROUBLED WATERS: THE CONTROL CYCLE

The Control Cycle, illustrated in **Figure 4**, represents the relationship between a Phase and the Phase that is two positions after it in the cycle. The initial Phase both supports and harnesses—or controls—the second succeeding Phase.

Figure 4. The Control Cycle

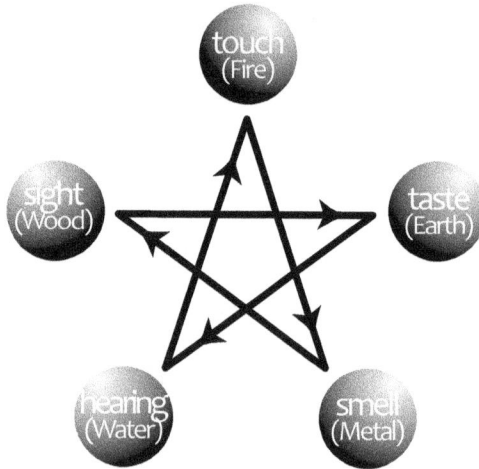

An excess of the initial Phase can lead to its overcontrol of the second succeeding Phase, thereby harming or diminishing the second one's functions. Should this be the case, the best solution is to sedate the first, excessive Phase, and tonify the overcontrolled, second Phase.

If Wood Overcontrols Earth: When Wood is excessive, it can overcontrol and impede Earth, for example, when anger causes stomach pain. **Solution**: Sedate Wood; tonify Earth.

If Fire Overcontrols Metal: When Fire is excessive, it can overcontrol and impede Metal. An example is when a sudden shock brings on an asthma attack.

Solution: Sedate Fire; tonify Metal.

If Earth Overcontrols Water: When Earth is excessive, it can overcontrol and impede Water. In this case, anxiety may, over time, deplete the Kidney Essence. **Solution**: Sedate Earth; tonify Water.

If Metal Overcontrols Wood: When Metal is excessive, it can overcontrol and impede Wood. An example of this is when a loss triggers rage or a seizure disorder. **Solution**: This relationship may be problematic within the Five-Phase theory to the degree that Wood, or the hyperactive Liver Yang associated with anger, does not become deficient. In this case, one might wish to sedate Metal, but perhaps not tonify Wood.

If Water Overcontrols Fire: When Water is excessive, it can overcontrol and impede Fire. An example of possible sequelae of this overcontrol: The *Staphlyococcinum* miasm with its tendency to chronic dysentery, abscess, and muco-purulent discharge, represents excessive Kidney. This, in turn, impedes the Heart, causing a susceptibility to endocarditis, frequent weeping, and aggravation from consolation. **Solution**: Because pathology of the Kidney is predominantly about deficiency, this relationship, too, may be problematic within the Five-Phase theory. Here one might want to tonify Fire but not sedate Water.

SHALLOW WATERS: THE COMPENSATION CYCLE

According to symptoms defined by sense-dimension theory, we may observe a cycle of relationships, called in TCM lore, the Insult Cycle. This cycle of relationships moves in a reverse direction, and is characterized not by an excess, but by a deficiency in an initial Phase, which leads to a fierce, compensatory excess in the second succeeding Phase. As such, this inverted cycle can be called the Compensation Cycle; it is depicted in **Figure 5** on the following page.

Insufficient control by the Phases in this cycle does not fully capture the compensatory dynamic at play here. The inverted movement and deficiency/excess, negative/positive force of this cycle produces such an extreme or perverse version of the positive pole of the core issue of the second succeeding sense dimension that it becomes a pitiful parody of the positive pole.

Below are descriptions of Compensation Cycle Phases and disorders. Homeopathic remedies in particular provide qualitatively detailed treatment strategies to cope with the powerful force and symptoms of the Phases of this cycle. Keep in mind that the central idea of each of these Phase relationships and their remedies also simultaneously overflows, flavors, and may perturb, the symptoms in the other Phases of the cycle.

Figure 5. The Compensation Cycle

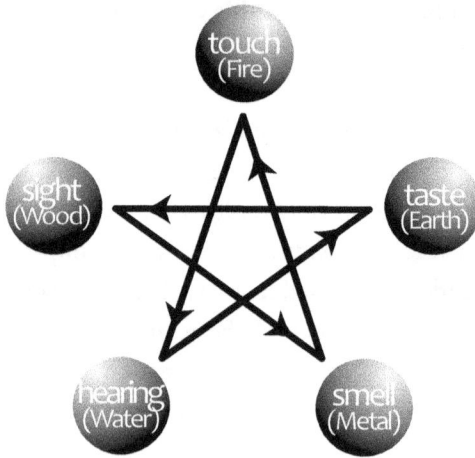

"Deficient Fire (Touch, Isolation, Heart) is compensated by → Excess Metal (Smell, Morbid Centeredness, Lungs)"

The key issues of the relationship between these two Phases are solipsism, which parodies in an intensely negative way the positive force of centeredness, and inauthenticity. The homeopathic remedies, Helleborus and Thuja, are indicated to treat the symptoms of these key issues.

Helleborus: "Hear No Evil, See No Evil"

The psychological profile of a person who is a solipsist is that of someone who is so depressed and shut down that the senses are dulled, and stupefaction and indifference set in. With Helleborus, indifference serves to compensate for isolation, often precipitated by a heartbreak.

Thuja: "I Cannot Access My Self-interest"

An inauthentic person is out of touch with his own self-interest. He may exhibit aspects of slavish conformism, artificial niceness, and falsity of self while harboring feelings of being unlovable, inner ugliness, hatred of his body, guilt, and shame. He may also have a delusion that his soul has been separated from his body. The radical disjunct is that social acceptance of the false self confirms that the authentic self is unacceptable. Thuja's most striking physical symptoms relate to skin pathologies, particularly the appearance of odd or mushroom-shaped warts.

In my practice I have found that about six weeks after a patient has taken a constitutional dose of Thuja, his more obvious symptoms may have been ameliorated, but significant depression may then be exposed. Peeling away the Thuja layer reveals the underlying trauma. If the patient is now strong enough to confront the trauma, Natrum sulphuricum, one of Thuja's complementary remedies, is indicated.

"Deficient Earth (Taste, Anxiety, Spleen) is compensated by $\longrightarrow$ Excess Water (Hearing, Morbid Consolidation, Kidneys)"

Stubbornness and self-consciousness are the two key issues governing the relationship between these Compensation Cycle Phases. The homeopathic remedy Silica is indicated for treatment of this Phase relationship.

Silica: "I Have Many Questions, But Won't Answer Even One of Yours" or "If I Speak Up, Everyone Will See Me"

Normally we think of stubborn individuals as being thick-skinned. A Silica person, however, has a tendency to be self-conscious and hypersensitive, yet, at the same time, rutted in stubbornness. In this Compensation Cycle relationship, pathological stubbornness reflects compensation for an overwhelming anxiety arising from a hypersensitivity so profound that the smallest of details and the most insignificant of slights will set him off.

"Deficient Metal (Smell, Disorientation, Lungs) is compensated by ⟶ Excess Wood (Sight, Morbid Creativity, Liver)"

The key issue in this Phase relationship is exhibitionism, for which the homeopathic remedy Hyoscyamus is indicated.

Hyoscyamus: "Gaze Upon My Shame"

"Warped inspiration" might be the term to use to characterize this condition. As a result of having had, for example, a harshly repressive childhood, an individual might become disoriented in the world of mature adults, and succumb to the attractions of immature, child-like people and behaviors. She might be an exhibitionist, act out inappropriate sexuality, become paranoiac, or fly into rages.

"Deficient Water (Hearing, Entropy, Kidneys) is compensated by ⟶ Excess Fire (Touch, Morbid Synchrony, Heart)"

The key issues here of codependency and dysrhythmia are treated by the remedies Arsenicum album and Tarentula hispanica.

Arsenicum album: "Unto Death, My Love"

The psychological profile of a codependent person is that of someone with an abnormal, overextended care for the welfare of friends and family. This codependency is rooted in an entropic lack of self-identity and in an anxiety related to an underlying sense and fear of impending death, involving either the self or the other. The individual may experience this physically as chilling or as burning heat within the body.

Tarentula hispanica: "I Dance to the Beat of My Own Drum"

Dysrhythmia associated with this Compensating-phase relationship may best be treated with the homeopathic remedy Tarentula hispanica, derived from the Spanish spider. Morbid synchrony here manifests as a disordered rhythm in the electrical activity of the heart; abnormal, rapid, rhythmic movements of the body; an aversion to being touched; palpitations; hyperactivity; impulsiveness; restlessness; and a need to hurry other people.

The patient's relationships may also lack a normal rhythm, alternating between dependency and possessiveness and shifting rapidly from flight to fight. The patient may have a great affinity for percussive music, dancing, horseback riding, and sexual activity.

The symptoms of deficiency in the Water Phase present as despair, melancholy, wildness, and incontinence.

"Deficient Wood (Sight, Chaos, Liver) is compensated by ⟶ Excess Earth (Taste, Morbid Challenge, Spleen)"

The key issue in this compensatory Phase relationship is recklessness, which may be treated homeopathically with the remedy Medorrhinum.

Medorrhinum: "Sex, Drugs, Extreme Sports"

A Medorrhinum person walks close to the edge, regardless of the danger involved. Passionate, driven, and obsessive about his interests, he may be attracted to sex, drugs, or extreme sports, and indifferent to anything outside his central focus. He tends towards wanting "all or nothing at all," to burning the candle at both ends.

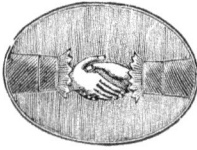

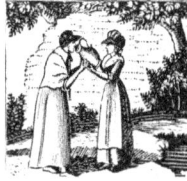

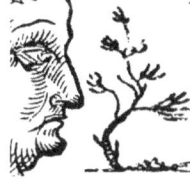

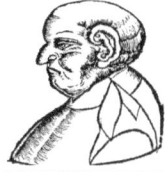

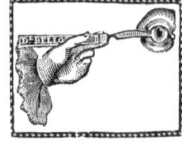

CHAPTER TEN

CREATE YOUR OWN FIVE SENSE DIMENSIONAL MANDALA

THE FIVE SENSE DIMENSIONS: CREATING A PERSONAL MANDALA

In this chapter you will build your own personal mandala for meditation, using the distinctive features of the positive and negative core issues of each of the five sense dimensions, and the cycles described in Chapter 9, "Encountering Charybdis: The Chronic Illness Vortex." A sense dimensional mandala template as well as specific questions about each of the core issues and cycles has been provided for you to guide you in creating and using your own mandala.

The Sanskrit word "mandala" has been translated to mean "circle." Although the mandala you will create here will be built on the foundation of the five circles of the Five-Phases Pentagram described in Chapter 2, "Beyond Biomedicine" with its corresponding five sense dimensions of touch, taste, smell, hearing, and sight, the intention of the mandala is to eventually create in you an awareness of the unity and oneness of body, mind, and spirit. Following the Generating Cycle of the five sense dimensions, you will eventually come full circle and produce a diagram on which you can meditate and potentially find healing of the self. Creating this mandala will require that you give open and honest answers to the questions relating to each of the sense dimensional core issues and a willingness to acknowledge and accept the diagrammatic picture of the self that emerges.

SENSE DIMENSIONAL MANDALA TEMPLATE
The Five Senses and Core Issues
(Based on the Generating Cycle)

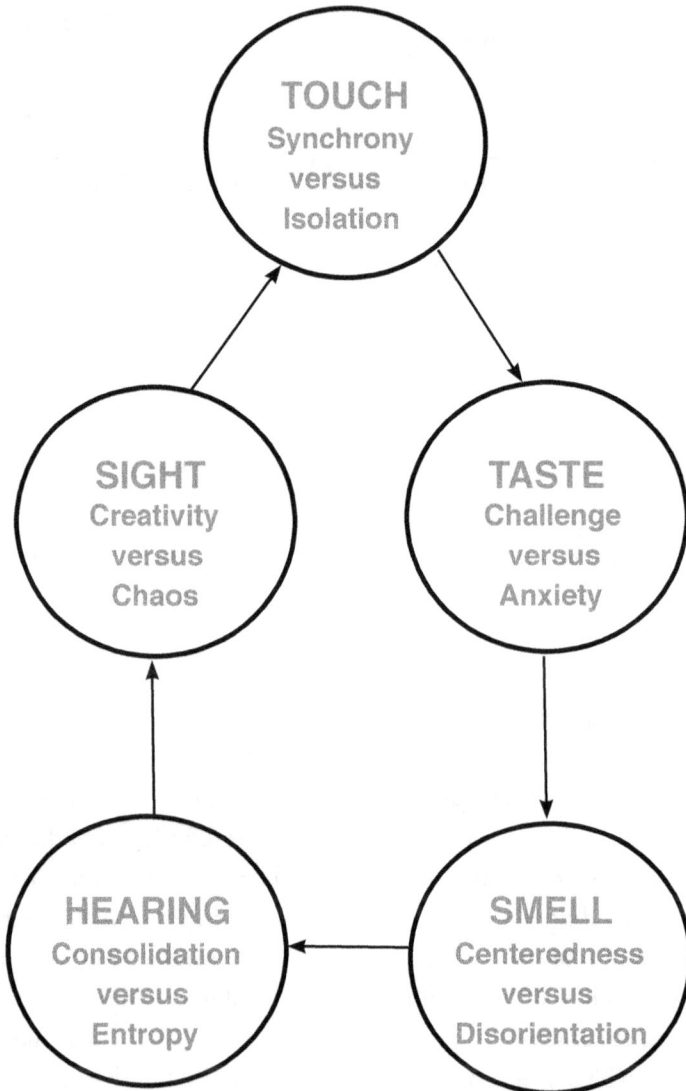

TOUCH
Synchrony
versus
Isolation

SIGHT
Creativity
versus
Chaos

TASTE
Challenge
versus
Anxiety

HEARING
Consolidation
versus
Entropy

SMELL
Centeredness
versus
Disorientation

YOUR PERSONAL MANDALA

(Fill circles by answering questions and following the
pattern of the Sense Dimensional Mandala Template)

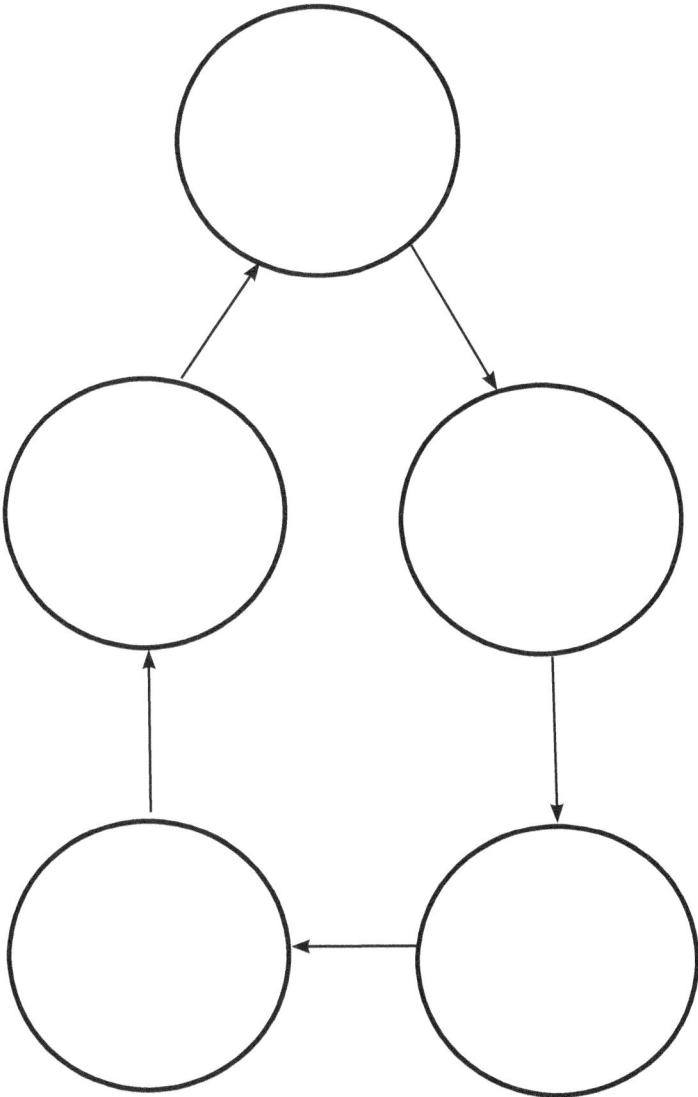

HEALING MEDITATION: THE
SENSE DIMENSIONAL MANDALA

CREATING YOUR PERSONAL MANDALA

By following the pattern of the Sense Dimensional Mandala Template, you will now create Your Personal Mandala. As shown, Your Personal Mandala consists of five blank circles that correspond to the circles and movement described in the Sense Dimension Mandala Template. To create your own mandala, you will go step by step, from circle to circle and sense dimension to sense dimension, in the direction indicated, and fill these circles with meaningful content based on your answers to the questions provided below for each of the sense dimensions. After answering each of the questions in the sense dimensions and filling in your mandala with answers, you will then assess and meditate on the results.

FIRST CIRCLE: THE DIMENSION OF TOUCH
SYNCHRONY VERSUS ISOLATION

A) Answer Questions About The Touch Dimension

1) **Ask yourself, to what extent am** I in *synchrony?*
   - What is the quality and depth of my close relationships?
   - How do I feel about, and act toward, those outside my immediate circle?
   - Am I passionate, joyful, spontaneous?
   - Does my anger blow over quickly?
   - Am I empathic, basically trustful?
   - Do I engage in philanthropy?
   - Do I enjoy physical intimacy?
   - Are my social encounters and activities rhythmic; that is, are they a comfortable give and take?
   - Is there a joyful practice of some sort in my life—yoga, singing, dance, poetry, drumming, playing a musical instrument?
   - Do I often cry or laugh?
   - Do I have a capacity for ecstasy?
   - Do I feel connected to my origins?
   - Is my awareness of a higher power or spiritual force operant?
   - Do I experience prayer as a call and response dynamic?

2) Ask yourself, to what extent am I in *isolation*?

- Were there bonding issues with my mother during my infancy?
- Am I estranged from my family or friends?
- Do I too often feel alone, unsupported, alienated?
- Do I feel that I have lost my way, my connection to God, or a source of spiritual power?
- Am I prone to circular thinking, and have a hard time getting out of my own way?
- Do I lack joy, frequently frown, have difficulty laughing or crying?
- Do I brood, sulk, or despair?
- Am I touch-deprived or touch-averse?
- Am I mistrustful or cynical?
- Am I prone to feelings of panic?
- Can my emotions fluctuate wildly?
- Do I experience heart palpitations or arrhythmia?
- Is my sleep disturbed?
- Do I frequently become feverish?

B) Fill In The Touch Dimension Circle

Fill in the sense dimension of touch circle with your most emotionally charged answers. Short phrase answers, such as "am joyous," or "am mistrustful" will suffice. Study your answers, and then convert them into an image or metaphor that captures your relation to the dimension of touch. Caption your circle with this image or metaphor. Now assess your response and decide: To what extent have I successfully resolved *synchrony versus isolation*?

If *synchrony* is my dominant pole, circle the word *synchrony*, and, depending on the degree of dominance, place one or more plus signs above the word. If *isolation* is my dominant pole, circle the word *isolation*, and depending on the degree of negativity, place one or more minus signs over the word.

SECOND CIRCLE: THE DIMENSION OF TASTE CHALLENGE VERSUS ANXIETY

A) Answer Questions About The Taste Dimension

1) Ask yourself, to what extent do I embrace *challenge*?

- Am I ambitious?
- Do I have a zest for life?
- Have I set meaningful goals for myself?
- Do I exercise regularly?
- When exercising do I ever push myself beyond my usual limits?
- Do I eat a nutritious diet utilizing local foods?
- Do I cook with care and artistry, chew my food thoroughly, favor home cooking over fast foods?
- Am I willing to experience hunger as well as satiety?
- Do I appreciate my parents, as well as earth-bound values such as the comforts of home, familial warmth, and contentedness?

2) Ask yourself, to what extent do I suffer from *anxiety*?

- Do I date many of my life issues to my childhood and adolescence?
- Am I perpetually nervous or overly self-conscious?
- Am I prone to sentimentality or overly aware of the needs of others?
- Do I often fell powerless, ineffective, immature, or insignificant?
- Am I easily intimidated or overpowered by others?
- Am I worshipful of domineering individuals or ideologies?
- Do I ever feel I am the victim of social, economic, or biological forces?
- Do I detest public speaking?
- Do I need to be in control, or do I lose myself in small details?
- Do I ever "bite off more than I can chew?"
- Am I ever tyrannical or bullying toward others?
- Am I intolerant of mistakes or defects?
- Am I prone to appetite or eating disorders?
- Do I suffer from heartburn, acid reflux, irritable bowel syndrome, or any other form of gastrointestinal distress?
- Am I often exhausted?
- Do my joints hurt?
- Am I sensitive to dampness?

B) Fill In The Taste Dimension Circle

Fill in the sense dimension of taste circle with your most emotionally charged answers. Short phrase answers, such as "love a challenge," and "bring it on!" or "hate confrontation" will suffice. Study your answers, and then convert them into an image or metaphor that captures your relation to the dimension of taste. Caption your circle with this image or metaphor. Now assess your response and decide: To what extent have I successfully resolved *challenge versus anxiety*?

If *challenge* is my dominant pole, circle the word *challenge*, and, depending on the degree of dominance, place one or more plus signs above the word. If *anxiety* is my dominant pole, circle the word *anxiety*, and depending on the degree of negativity, place one or more minus signs over the word.

THIRD CIRCLE: THE DIMENSION OF SMELL
CENTEREDNESS VERSUS DISORIENTATION

A) Answer Questions About The Smell Dimension

1) Ask yourself, to what extent am I *centered*?
- Do I retain my composure under stress?
- Can I adapt to necessary change?
- Do I live in the moment?
- I my sense of time strong?
- When confronted with loss, am I able to grieve to completion and move on?
- Do I have a strong sense of my identity both within my family and in the world?
- Is meditation part of my regular practice?
- Can I think strategically?
- Is my memory sharp?
- Do I practice martial arts or strategic games, such as chess?
- Do I, or would I, like to go sailing?
- Do I avoid scent pollution?
- Do I value clean air?
- Is my stamina good?
- Do I "know which way the wind blows?"

2) Ask yourself, to what extent am I *disoriented*?

- Do I fluster easily?
- Do I resist change?
- Is it difficult for me to overcome loss?
- Do I tend to cry in private?
- Am I often sad for no particular reason?
- When my feelings are hurt do I try to hide my pain from those around me?
- Am I prone to nostalgia or déjà vu?
- Is my memory or sense of direction poor?
- Is my sense of time poor?
- Do I suffer from food or airborne allergies?
- Is it sometimes difficult for me to swallow?
- Am I often congested?
- Do I gasp, wheeze, or become short of breath?
- Is my skin excessively dry?
- Do I break out in a rash when stressed?

B) Fill In The Taste Dimension Circle

Fill in the sense dimension of smell circle with your most emotionally charged answers. Short phrase answers, such as "am highly composed," or "am overly self-conscious" will suffice. Study your answers, and then convert them into an image or metaphor that captures your relation to the dimension of smell. Caption your circle with this image or metaphor. Now assess your response and decide: To what extent have I successfully resolved *centeredness versus disorientation*?

If *centeredness* is my dominant pole, circle the word *centeredness*, and, depending on the degree of dominance, place one or more plus signs above the word. If *disorientation* is my dominant pole, circle the word *disorientation*, and depending on the degree of negativity, place one or more minus signs over the word.

FOURTH CIRCLE: THE DIMENSION OF HEARING CONSOLIDATION VERSUS ENTROPY

A) Answer Questions About The Hearing Dimension

1) Ask yourself, to what extent am I *consolidated*?

- Do I practice moderation in work, recreation, diet, and sexual activity?
- Am I vigilant in securing my family's needs with regard to safety, food, and shelter?
- Do I have a sense of the significance of my own life?
- Does my work provide me with a mission or reflect a calling?
- Am I concerned with my legacy?
- Is the improvement of my community a matter of importance to me?
- Do I maintain good body heat?
- Are my bones and teeth strong?

2) Ask yourself, to what extent am I subject to *entropy*?

- Am I generally fearful?
- Do I obsess about death?
- Do I feel that life has no meaning?
- Do I vacillate between extremes?
- Am I an "all or nothing" person?
- Has anyone ever referred to me as a "Jekyll and Hyde?"
- Does my mind go around in circles?
- Do I feel that I am surrounded by enemies?
- Do I exercise poor judgment in my choice of partners?
- Can it feel as if everything is falling apart around me?
- At times, am I deeply depressed or alienated from society?
- Are diseases such as tuberculosis, syphilis, gonorrhea, cancer, or heart disease notable among my parents, grandparents, or great-grandparents?
- Is there a family history of alcoholism or drug abuse?
- Am I myself susceptible to alcoholism?
- Do I possess an addictive personality?
- Are my teeth vulnerable to decay?
- Do I suffer from osteopenia or osteoporosis?
- Is my bladder ever troublesome?
- Do I have one or more genetic ailments?

B) Fill In The Hearing Dimension Circle

Fill in the sense dimension of hearing circle with your most emotionally charged answers. Short phrase answers, such as "have moderate lifestyle," or "am overindulgent" will suffice. Study your answers, and then convert them into an image or metaphor that captures your relation to the dimension of hearing. Caption your circle with this image or metaphor. Now assess your response and decide: To what extent have I successfully resolved *consolidation versus entropy*?

If *consolidation* is my dominant pole, circle the word *consolidation*, and, depending on the degree of dominance, place one or more plus signs above the word. If *entropy* is my dominant pole, circle the word *entropy*, and depending on the degree of negativity, place one or more minus signs over the word.

FIFTH CIRCLE: THE DIMENSION OF SIGHT
CREATIVITY VERSUS CHAOS

A) Answer Questions About The Sight Dimension

1) Ask yourself, to what extent am I *creative*?
- Do I follow a creative pursuit such as painting, drawing, landscaping, or playing a musical instrument?
- Can I keep things in perspective?
- Am I objective?
- Do I clearly and cleanly attend to detail?
- Do I experience "flow" in my activities?
- Can I convert my anger into creative action?
- Do I appreciate color, design, or precision?
- Do I value simplicity?
- Do I avoid clutter?
- Am I able to see the "big picture?"
- Is it possible for me to think like a world citizen or like a visionary?

2) Ask yourself, to what extent am I subject to *chaos*?

- Am I overly judgmental or prone to bias or prejudice?
- Do I adhere rigidly to my beliefs?
- Is it difficult for me to accept change?
- Is it hard for me to make up my mind?
- Do I harbor resentment, rage, grudges, or bitterness?
- Can I lash out blindly?
- Has anyone remarked on my possessiveness?
- Am I overly materialistic?
- Do I tend to hoard?
- Do I lack the ability to organize my life?
- Am I prone to have headaches or visual disorders?
- Do I stutter or stammer?
- Are my ligaments and muscles stiff?
- Am I twitchy, restless, or subject to seizures?
- Do I suffer from any circulatory ailments?
- If a woman, are my periods painful or irregular?
- Do I have infertility issues?

B) Fill In The Sight Dimension Circle

Fill in the sense dimension of sight circle with your most emotionally charged answers. Short phrase answers, such as "am objective," or "am a rageaholic" will suffice. Study your answers, and then convert them into an image or metaphor that captures your relation to the dimension of sight. Caption your circle with this image or metaphor. Now assess your response and decide: To what extent have I successfully resolved *creativity versus chaos*?

If *creativity* is my dominant pole, circle the word *creativity*, and, depending on the degree of dominance, place one or more plus signs above the word. If *chaos* is my dominant pole, circle the word *chaos*, and depending on the degree of negativity, place one or more minus signs over the word.

EVALUATING AND LEARNING FROM YOUR RESPONSES

After having completed the exercises, proceeding step-by-step through each of the sense dimensions in the Generating Cycle and assigning positive or negative values to the core issue of each sense dimension, you can now evaluate your responses. If you gave candid and open answers to the questions and allowed yourself to form a general impression of where you stand in relation to each sense dimension's core issue, you should have had little trouble in assigning unambiguous positive and negative values.

THE GENERATING CYCLE

In an ideal state of health, your Personal Mandala would express positive values for all five sense dimensions within a Generating Cycle. As you move forward clockwise in the Generating Cycle, keep in mind that the positive, successful resolution of the core issues in one sense dimension helps to promote the positive, successful resolution of the core issue in the succeeding sense dimension.

If you find that a particular sense dimension is charged equally with positive and negative values so that you cannot decide which pole of the core issue is dominant, you may do one or both of the following:

1) Emphasize that this sense dimension has a problem by drawing another, larger circle around the sense dimension's circle on the mandala; this will draw your attention to the inflamed nature of this sense dimension's core issue and will encourage you to address the issue.

2) Use both the positive and negative values! Create two alternative mandalas, one mandala giving this sense dimension issue a positive value, and the other mandala giving the issue a negative value. By comparing the two, you may be able to decide that one of the sense dimensional models is more accurate than the other, but you may also find that both models contribute to your self-understanding.

USE THE MOTHER-CHILD RELATIONSHIPS

As described in Chapter 9, "Encountering Charybdis: The Chronic Illness Vortex," as you proceed clockwise in the Generating Cycle around the mandala, from one sense dimension to the next, each sense dimension has the property of generating or giving energy to the next succeeding one. This pairing relationship is known in TCM as the "Mother-Child" relationship, in which each phase of the Generating Cycle is "Mother" to the next succeeding phase, the "Child." If you encounter a negative value in a sense dimension, go back one circle to the preceding sense dimension, the Mother, and look carefully at its nurturing relationship to the Child and the Child's negative value. Think about and meditate on what state of being or activities within the Mother might be used to help resolve the negative value within the Child. Examine carefully, too, whether the negative Child is too strong or too demanding in relation to a weaker Mother, in which case think about and meditate on how you can tonify or support the Mother and sedate or drain the excessive quality of the dominant Child and help resolve the Child's negative core issue.

OTHER CYCLES: RETROGRADE GENERATING, CONTROL, AND COMPENSATION

In addition to the Generating Cycle, Chapter 9, "Encountering Charybdis: The Chronic Illness Vortex" describes and pictures in detail three other energy cycles and how you can be affected by them. If you wish to go more deeply into an analysis of the sense dimension core issues in your Personal Mandala you can take into consideration some of the effects of these other cycles. What matters most, however, is that you engage with your Personal Mandala as a whole, using it in the most creative way you can as a tool for self-investigation and healing.

Briefly, the three cycles other than the Generating Cycle either move in an inverted direction from clockwise or affect issues that do not directly follow, but are two circles removed, from a given sense dimension. These differences can impact the dynamics of the relationships between the sense dimensions and their core issues.

THE RETROGRADE GENERATING CYCLE

On the whole, the four cycles are not mutually exclusive, meaning that they can operate simultaneously, the major exception being the Generating Cycle and the Retrograde Generating Cycle. Because energy in the Retrograde Generating Cycle moves counterclockwise in a reverse pattern from the Generating Cycle, these two cycles cannot function at the same time. In the inverted pattern of the Retrograde Generating Cycle, the negative pole of one sense dimension so aggressively brings out the negative pole of the next sense dimension, that it may produce a severe pathology.

You may identify a Retrograde Generating Cycle by the appearance of intensely negative values appearing in two or more successive sense dimensions. Although it may be useful to study and meditate on this energetic inversion, it is likely urgent in this situation that you seek medical attention either from a physician or from a qualified acupuncturist or homeopath.

THE CONTROL CYCLE

If you have identified a negative value in a sense dimension and have gone back one circle, as previously described, and looked at the "Mother" in the sense dimension immediately preceding, you will discover that this initial sense dimension also has a slightly dominating influence over the sense dimension that is two circles ahead of it in the cycle. This relationship which involves two circles or stations between sense dimensions is called the Control Cycle, and it is normally supportive or controlling. If, however, the initial sense dimension is inordinately controlling or overly dominant of the second succeeding sense dimension, the second one's functions can be negatively influenced, harmed, or diminished, and disharmony occurs. Again, meditate on this relationship and think about activities that might reduce the excessive dominance of the initial sense dimension and support the resolution of the core issue of the sense dimension two circles ahead.

THE COMPENSATION CYCLE

Known in TCM as the Insult Cycle, the Compensation Cycle is characterized by a reversal in direction of movement around the cycle and a deficiency in the initial sense dimension that leads to an excess in the sense dimension two circles after it. The specific interactions between the phases within the Compensation Cycle are described in detail in Chapter 9, "Encountering Charybdis: The Chronic Illness Vortex."

In the Compensation Cycle, as the dominator/dominated relationship inverts so does the positive/negative relationship. What is particularly forceful about the Compensation Cycle is its element of perverseness, in which a positive value of a sense dimension can be manifested in such an extremely compensatory way that it becomes a parody of that value. For example, in the inverted Compensation Cycle, an inability to control one's anxiety (sense dimension of taste) is compensated for by a morbid consolidation (sense dimension of hearing) that is expressed by excessive self-consciousness or self-absorption (compressed or consolidated "self-ness").

Once you have recognized this compensatory dynamic, you may evaluate its utility to you as well as its liability in terms of your susceptibility to illness. Think about and meditate on the compensation dynamics within the controlling sense dimension. If you have the option, you may consult a homeopath who is able to understand these dynamics and prescribe appropriate remedies.

FURTHER SUGGESTIONS FOR USE OF YOUR PERSONAL MANDALA

Once you have spent sufficient time charting, studying, periodically updating, and meditating on, your Personal Mandala, your mandala will yield an individualized portrait of mind, body, and health that can also serve to chart spiritual progress. You can also embellish your mandala with personally selected poetry and visual imagery.

Another application of the mandala that has the potential to serve spiritual development is in the enhancement of the marriage relationship. For the purpose of expanding mutual empathy, if both partners have created Personal Mandalas and have an honest and open relationship with each other, each may then attempt, by using their mandalas, to develop an ever deeper comprehension of the mind, body, and spirit of the Other.

In a perhaps more empirical version of the same dynamic, each partner could also work under the direction of a qualified homeopath to undertake a mild proving of his or her own and the partner's constitutional remedies best suited to resolve issues revealed by the mandalas.

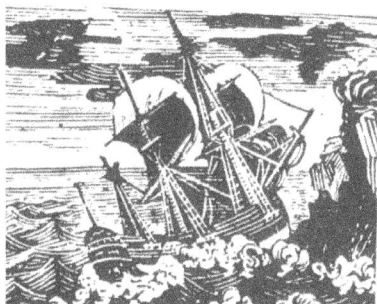

EPILOGUE
TURNING OUR GREAT SHIP

THE VOYAGE HOME

If you have absorbed and applied some of the novel concepts about the five sense dimensions and chronic illness offered in this book, you may be well on your way to turning the Great Ship—our human form—toward the health-giving, pristine energy of the Self, our true home.

In this epilogue you will find a table that brings together in a comprehensive matrix the juxtaposition of the five sense dimensions with the elements of Traditional Chinese Medicine. The table can stand alone or serve as a quick reference tool as you read through the book or when you create your Personal Mandala.

Transformation can feel so natural as to appear uncaused. A patient may be oblivious that anything has actually changed, in which case a practitioner receives scant acknowledgement for a desirable outcome, even when it takes place with suddenness.

My favorite example of obliviousness concerns an intense and angry fifty-year-old woman who sought me out for homeopathic care. "Can you do anything for me?" she pleaded. "All I want to do is work. I work sixty-hour weeks regularly and have no interest in ever taking a vacation. I want nothing to do with my husband. I have a son, living in Portugal, but I have no interest in seeing him. Can you help me?"

My prescription for her was a single, 200c dose of the homeopathic remedy

Nux vomica. Within several weeks I picked up a phone message in which she asked to cancel her appointment for a follow-up session. When I phoned her back, she said, "I'm not coming in because I'm the same." When I asked her about details concerning her experience while she was on the remedy, she replied, "Well, I mean, I'm fine. But why shouldn't I be? My husband and I decided to take a vacation—six months earlier than we had originally planned—to go visit our son in Portugal. So why shouldn't I feel fine?"

My office at the time was on the second floor of a building complex which also had a large room on the first floor that was used for yoga classes. Soon after the phone conversation took place, I was passing by the open door of the class on my way up to my office when I saw my former patient sitting in the class in one of the relaxed yoga postures.

Reflecting back on this case, it occurs to me how perfectly it expresses the radical disjunct that is unique to health care practitioners. Though wishing to effect a change in our clients, perhaps when change is least recognized that we best succeed.

> *Our Great Ship—our human form—is built of dreams, physical and emotional needs, and unique capabilities, fashioned to withstand life's squalls, gales, and treacherous currents. The Sea of Life on which our Great Ship sails has also been given to us as a source of primal life energy.*
>
> *A ship at sea and the wide sea maintain a tenuous relationship. A ship is buoyed, and the sea yields up its bountiful life for the sailors; yet often trade winds and perfect storms buffet the ship and destroy it. Like a ship at sea, our Great Ship endures life's volatility and discovers that the Sea of Life is neither unlimited nor unconditionally ours.*
>
> *In this book I have offered a new model to redirect our Great Ship, measure for measure, toward the health-giving, primal energy of the Sea of Life.*

The Five Sense Dimensions and
Traditional Chinese Medicine

Sense	TOUCH	TASTE	SMELL	HEARING	SIGHT
System	Circulation	Metabolism	Respiration	Reproduction	Neurological
Organ	Heart	Spleen/ Stomach	Lung	Kidneys	Liver
Phase	Fire	Earth	Metal	Water	Wood
Illness	Transient symptoms	Acute symptoms	Periodic symptoms	Susceptibilities Addictions Inherited disorders	Chronic illnesses
Function	Safety	Conformism	Strategy	Integration	Breakthrough
Core Dilemma	Synchrony/ Isolation (Terror)	Challenge/ Anxiety (Worry)	Centeredness/ Disorientation (Abandonment)	Consolidation/ Entropy (Awe)	Creativity/ Chaos (Anger)
Associated Interventions	Trauma care Massage Sculpture	Nutrition Exercise Culinary arts Gardening	Acupuncture Martial arts Chess Aromatherapy	Qi gong Yoga Twelve Steps Music Chanting	Homeopathy (Constitutional) Visual arts Writing
Stage of Life	Childhood	Adolescence	Adulthood	Middle Age	Old Age/ Regeneration
Taste	Bitter	Sweet	Umami	Salty	Sour
Sound Quality	Rhythm	Harmonics	Timbre	Pitch	Intensity
Season	Summer	Indian Summer	Fall	Winter	Spring

NOTES

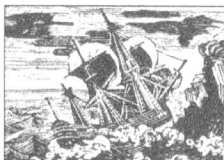

CHAPTER ONE
TURNING OUR GREAT SHIP: A SEA CHANGE

1. The quote is widely known as "Maslow's Maxim" or "Maslow's Hammer." http://www.abraham-maslow.com/m_motivation/Maslows_Hammer.asp. Accessed October 30, 2009.

2. *Ralph Waldo Emerson Journals* (published 1904 to 1914). The ten-volume Edward Emerson edition of the *Journals*, originally published in Boston by Houghton Mifflin, from 1904 through 1914, contains more than 5,000 pages of material. The originals are housed at the Houghton Library at Harvard University and cover the period between 1820, when Emerson was a Junior at Harvard, and 1876, when Emerson stopped writing in his journals.

3. This *koan* can be found among the hundred *koans* of the *Hekiganroku*, or *Blue Cliff Record*, a collection of Chán Buddhist *koans* compiled in China during the Song dynasty, in the 12th century CE. http://perso.ens-lyon.fr/eric.boix/Koan/Hekiganroku/index.html. Accessed November 1, 2009.

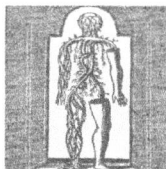

CHAPTER TWO
BEYOND BIOMEDICINE

1. Kaptchuk T. *The Web That Has No Weaver: Understanding Chinese Medicine.* New York, NY: Congdon and Weed; 1983.

2. Young A. *The Reflexive Universe: Evolution of Consciousness.* San Francisco, CA: Delacorte Press; 1976:273-274.

3. Daniel C. Dennett, D.Phil., the author of *Breaking the Spell* (Viking, 2006), *Freedom Evolves* (Viking Penguin, 2003), and *Darwin's Dangerous Idea* (Simon &Schuster, 1995), is university professor and Austin B. Fletcher Professor of Philosophy, and Co-Director of the Center for Cognitive Studies at Tufts University, Medford, MA.

4. Frankl V. *Man's Search for Meaning: An Introduction to Logotherapy.* London, England: Hodder & Stoughton; 1959.

CHAPTER THREE
THE DIMENSION OF TOUCH

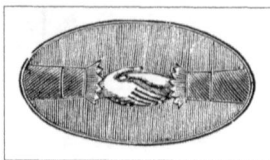

1. Hertenstein MJ, Holmes R, McCullough M. The communication of emotion via touch. *Emotion*. 2009;9:566-573.

2. Gick B, Derrick D. Aero-tactile integration in speech perception. *Nature*. 2009;462:502-504.

3. Strogatz S. *SYNC: The Emerging Science of Spontaneous Order*. New York, NY: Hyperion; 2003.

4. Kivimäki M, Ferrie JE, Brunner E, et al. Justice at work and reduced risk of coronary heart disease among employees: the Whitehall II study. *Archives of Internal Medicine*. 2005;165:2245-2251.

5. Mangialavori M. *Some Cactaceae in Homeopathic Medicine*. Wood B, Amiri B, eds. Notes from the 2005—11th Summer Seminar; Alghero, Italy. http://www.mangialavori.com/inglese/cactacee.htm. Accessed May 16, 2010.

6. Scholten J. *Homeopathy and the Elements*. Utrecht, The Netherlands: Stichting Alonnissos Publishing; 1996.

7. Scholten J. *Homeopathy and the Minerals*. Utrecht, The Netherlands: Stichting Alonnissos Publishing; 1993.

8. Scholten J. *Secret Lanthanides*. Utrecht, The Netherlands: Stichting Alonnissos Publishing; 2005.

9. 1996 Australian film, *Shine*, based on the life of the pianist David Helfgott.

10. Rice DP. The economic impact of schizophrenia. *J Clin Psychiatry*. 1999;60(suppl 1):4-6.

11. Wu EQ, Birnbaum HG, Shi L, Ball DE, Kessler RC, Moulis M, Aggarwal J. The economic burden of schizophrenia in the United States in 2002. *J Clin Psychiatry*. 2005;66:1122-1129.

12. Edward C. Whitmont,M.D., quoted in Vermeulen F. *Prisma: The Arcana of Materia Medica Illuminated: Similars and Parallels Between Substance and Remedy*. Haarlem, The Netherlands: Emryss b.v. Publishers; 2002:866.

13. Eaton W, Mortensen PB, Agerbo E, Byrne M, Mors O, Ewald H. Coeliac disease and schizophrenia: population based case control study with linkage of Danish national registers. *BMJ*. 2004;328:438-439.

14. West J, Logan RF, Hubbard RB, Card TR. Risk of schizophrenia in people with coeliac disease, ulcerative colitis and Crohn's disease: a general population-based study. *Aliment Pharmacol Ther*. 2006;23:71-74.

15. Ludvigsson JF, Osby U, Ekbom A, Montgomery SM. Coeliac disease and risk of schizophrenia and other general population cohort study. *Scand J Gastroenterol.* 2007;42:179-185.

16. Shan L, Molberg Ø, Parrot I, et al. Structural basis for gluten intolerance in celiac sprue. *Science.* 2002;297:2275-2279.

CHAPTER FOUR
THE DIMENSION OF TASTE

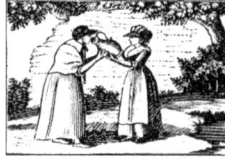

1. Bellisle F. Glutamate and the umami taste: sensory, metabolic, nutritional and behavioural considerations: a review of the literature published in the last 10 years. *Neurosci Biobehav Rev.* 1999;23:423-438.

2. Mizushige T, Inoue K, Fushiki T. Why is fat so tasty? chemical reception of fatty acid on the tongue. *J Nutr Sci Vitaminol.* 2007;53:1-4.

3. Khakh BS, Burnstock G. The double life of ATP in humans. *Scientific American.* 2009;301:84-92.

4. Schemann M. Control of gastrointestinal motility by the "gut brain" - the enteric nervous system. *J Pediatr Gastroenterol Nutr.* 2005;41:S4-S6.

5. Sankaran R. *The Substance of Homoeopathy: The Natural Classification of Drugs.* Bombay, India: Homoeopathic Medical Publishers; 1994:135.

6. Scholten J. *Homeopathy and the Elements.* Utrecht, The Netherlands: Stichting Alonnissos Publishing; 1996:350.

7. Moalem S, Storey KB, Percy ME, Peros MC, Perl DP. The sweet thing about type I diabetes: a cryoprotective evolutionary adaptation. *Med Hpotheses.* 2005;65:8-16.

8. Centers for Disease Control and Prevention. National diabetes fact sheet: national estimates and general information on diabetes and prediabetes in the United States, 2011. Atlanta, GA: U.S. Department of Health and Human Services, Centers for Disease Control and Prevention, 2011. NIH Publication No. 11-3892, February 2011. http://diabetes.niddk.nih.gov/dm/pubs/statistics/index.htm#fast. Accessed February 10, 2011.

9. The Weight-control Information Network (WIN). Overweight and obesity statistics. Bethesda, MD: National Institute of Diabetes and Digestive and Kidney Diseases, National Institutes of Health. NIH Publication No. 04-4158, updated February 2010. http://www.win.niddk.nih.gov/publications/PDFs/stat9042z.pdf. Accessed May 22, 2011.

10. Assilem MA. *The Mad Hatter's Tea Party.* Kandern, Germany: Narayana Verlag GmbH; 2002.

11. Robin Logan, quoted in Vermeulen F. *Prisma: The Arcana of Materia Medica Illuminated: Similars and Parallels Between Substance and Remedy*. Haarlem, The Netherlands: Emryss b.v. Publishers; 2002:772.

12. Although introduced within the context of mitochondrial dysfunction, the Graphites' state more accurately is associated with a deficiency of Liver blood caused by stagnation arising from frustration; this places Graphites within the dimension of sight, whose core conundrum pits creativity against chaos. The giveaways are that Graphites' nails (controlled by the Liver) tend to become thick and coarse, and the seizure disorders that are treated with Graphites manifest Wind or Chaos.

CHAPTER FIVE
THE DIMENSION OF SMELL

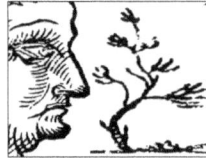

1. Bendesky A, Makoto T, Rockman MV, Kruglyak L, Bargmann CI. Catecholamine receptor polymorphisms affect decision-making in *C. elegans*. *Nature*. 2011;472:313-318. See also Wade N. In tiny worm, unlocking secrets of the brain. *The New York Times*. June 20, 2011:D1.

2. The Chinese alchemical treatise by Ge Hong (Ko Hung, 283—343 CE) claimed that drinking a potion with cinnabar, crystallized red mercuric sulfide, could make one immortal and carry one at will to the highest heaven. (For a complete translation of Ge Hong's "The Inner Chapters," see Ware JR. *Alchemy, Medicine and Religion in the China of A.D. 320: The Nei P'ien of Ko Hung*. New York, NY: Dover Publications, Inc.; 1981.)

3. This capability, known as chirality, did not become well-known until the 1980s, after gas chromatography had become sufficiently advanced to reliably identify and distinguish mirror-image (enantiomeric) chemicals. Chirality can be very simply defined as "handedness"; that is, the existence of left/right opposition or left-hand and right-hand mirror images. The term "chiral" is derived from the Greek name *kheir* meaning "hand"; it was apparently coined by Lord Kelvin, in 1904, in his "Baltimore Lectures on Molecular Dynamics and the Wave Theory of Light." (For a detailed discussion of chirality and odorants, see Leffingwell JC. Chirality & odour perception. 2002. http://www.leffingwell.com/chirality/chirality.htm. Accessed June 10, 2010.)

4. Although sound-quality characteristics such as pitch or volume relate directly to a sound wave itself, timbre is associated with the texture of the instrument in which a sound wave is produced and how the wave extends through, or is limited by, its medium; in other words, the sound wave's orientation to its surroundings. Themes within the

dimension of smell may shed light on certain voice disorders related to timbre.

5. Thanks to Karen Allen for initiating me into the importance of Imponderables.

6. alz.org, Alzheimer's Association Web site. Alzheimer's disease prevalence rates rise to more than five million in the United States. *Alzheimer News 3/20/2007.* http://www. alz.org/news_and_events_rates_rise.asp. Accessed June 11, 2010.

7. Kessels RP, de Haan EH, Kappelle LJ, Postma A. Varieties of human spatial memory: a meta-analysis on the effects of hippocampal lesions. *Brain Res Brain Res Rev.* 2001; 35:295-303.

8. Smith DM, Mizumori SJ. Hippocampal place cells, context, and episodic memory. *Hippocampus.* 2006;16:716-729.

9. Winocur G, Moscovitch M, Fogel S, Rosenbaum RS, Sekeres M. Preserved spatial memory after hippocampal lesions: effects of extensive experience in a complex environment. *Nat Neuosci.* 2005;8:273-275.)

10. National Institute on Aging, U.S. National Institutes of Health, National Advisory Council on Aging. Summary Minutes: The Eighty-Fourth Meeting; Bethesda, MD; September 24-25, 2001; Section V.

11. De Meyer G, Shapiro F, Vanderstichele H, et al. Diagnosis-independent Alzheimer disease biomarker signature in cognitively normal elderly people. *Arch Neuol.* 2010;67:949-956.

12. Liu L, Drouet V, Wu JW, et al. Trans-synaptic spread of tau pathology *in vivo.* *PLoS ONE.* 2012;7(2): e31302. doi:10.1371/journal.pone.0031302.

13. Cacabelos R, Fernandez-Novoa L, Lombardi V, Kubota Y, Takeda M. Molecular genetics of Alzheimer's disease and aging. *Methods Find Exp Clin Pharmacol.* 2005;27(suppl A): 1-573.

14. Finch CE. Evolution of the human lifespan and diseases of aging: roles of infection, inflammation, and nutrition. *PNAS.* 2010;107(suppl 1):1718-1724.

15. Gu Y, Nieves JW, Stern Y, Luchsinger JA, Scarmeas N. Food combination and Alzheimer disease risk: a protective diet. *Arch Neurol* [published online]. April 12, 2010(doi:10.1001/archneurol.2010.84). Accessed May 15, 2010.

16. De Filippo C, Cavalieri D, Di Paola M, et al. Impact of diet in shaping gut microbiota revealed by a comparative study in children from Europe and rural Africa. *Proc Natl Acad Sci U S A.* 2010;107:14691-14696.

17. Talamo BR, Rudel R, Kosik KS, et al. Pathological changes in olfactory neurons in patients with Alzheimer's disease. *Nature.* 1989; 337: 736-739.

18. The Taoists recognized five major flavors and associated each with an element or sense dimension, while Western understanding of flavor-receptivity noted only four flavors—sweet, sour, bitter, and salty. By confirming the existence of a fifth flavor, known as "umami," and its own specific tongue receptor cells for pungency, modern Western

knowledge has aligned itself with that of the ancient Chinese. (Chaudhari N, Pereira E, Roper SD. Taste receptors for umami: the case for multiple receptors. *Am J Clin Nutr.* 2009;90:738S-742S.)

19. Gambetti P, Kong Q, Zou W, Parchi P, Chen SG. Sporadic and familial CJD: classification and characterisation. *Br Med Bull.* 2003;66:213-239.

20. Prusiner SB. The prion diseases. *Sc Am.* 1995;272:48-51, 54-7. Review.

21. Seitz R, von Auer F, Blümel J, et al. Impact of vCJD on blood supply. *Biologicals.* 2007;35:79-97.

22. Kong Q, Zheng M, Casalone C, et al. Evaluation of the human transmission risk of an atypical bovine spongiform encephalopathy prion strain. *J Virol.* 2008;82:3697-3701.

23. Laurén J, Gimbel DA, Nygaard HB, Gilbert JW, Strittmatter SM. Cellular prion protein mediates impairment of synaptic plasticity by amyloid-beta oligomers. *Nature.* 2009;457:1128-1132.

24. Ghoshal N, Cali I, Perrin RJ, et al. Codistribution of amyloid beta plaques and spongiform degeneration in familial Creutzfeldt-Jakob disease with the E200K-129M hapolyte. *Arch Neurol.* 2009;66:1240-1246.

25. Meiner Z, Gabizon R, Prusiner SB. Familial Creutzfeldt-Jakob disease: codon 200 prion disease in Libyan Jews. *Medicine (Baltimore).* 1997;76:227-237.

26. Gigi A. The role of stress and anxiety in the onset of familial Creutzfeldt-Jakob disease (CJD): review. *Stress.* 2009;12:371-378.

27. Bland, JS. *Genetic Nutritioneering.* Keats Publishing: Los Angeles, CA.; 1999.

28. Wellcome Trust Sanger Institute Cancer Genome Project. Cancer gene census: cancer genes that have frameshift mutations. http://www.sanger.ac.uk/genetics/CGP/census/frameshift_mutation.shtml. Accessed April 5, 2010.

CHAPTER SIX
The Dimension of Hearing

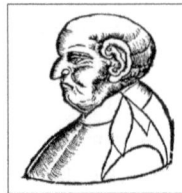

1. Hellinger B, Weber G, Beaumont H. *Love's Hidden Symmetry: What Makes Love Work in Relationships.* Phoenix, Ariz.: Zeig, Tucker & Theisen; 1998.

2. Carroll MP. *Catholic Cults and Devotions: A Psychological Inquiry.* Montreal, Canada: McGill-Queen's University Press; 1989:31.

3. Cohen S, Janicki-Deverts D, Miller G. Psychological stress and disease. *JAMA.* 2007;298:1685-1687.

4. NIDA Newsletter, National Institute of Drug Abuse (NIDA), National Institutes of Health, U.S. Department of Health and Human Services. Addiction: drugs, brains, and behavior—the science of addiction. NIH Publication No. 07-5605. Reprinted February 2008. http://www.drugabuse.gov/science of addiction. Accessed June 15, 2010.

5. Scholten J. *Secret Lanthanides*. Utrecht, The Netherlands: Stichting Alonnissos Publishing; 2005.

6. I am indebted to Jackie Clasen for bringing the Lanthanides tendency to addiction to my attention.

7. Emerman M, Malik HS. Paleovirology—modern consequences of ancient viruses. *PLoS Biol.* 2010;8(2):e1000301. doi:10.1371/journal.pbio.1000301.

8. Hajra S, Ghosh SK, Jayaram M. The centromere-specific histone variant Cse4p (CENP-A) is essential for functional chromatin architecture at the yeast 2-μm circle partitioning locus and promotes equal plasmid segregation. *J Cell Biol.* 2006;174:779-790.

9. Malik HS. A hitchhiker's guide to survival finally makes CENs. *J Cell Biol.* 2006;174:747-749.

10. National Kidney and Urologic Diseases Information Clearinghouse (NKU-DIC), A service of the National Institute of Diabetes and Digestive and Kidney Diseases (NIDDK), National Institutes of Health, U.S. Department of Health and Human Services. The kidneys and how they work. NIH Publication No. 09–3195. February 2009. http://kidney.niddk.nih.gov/kudiseases/pubs/yourkidney. Accessed June 20, 2010.

11. Vermeulen F. *Prisma: The Arcana of Materia Medica Illuminated: Similars and Parallels Between Substance and Remedy*. Haarlem, The Netherlands: Emryss b.v. Publishers; 2002:314.

12. The U.S. Department of Energy (DOE) Human Genome Project Information Web site genomics.energy.gov. Genetic disease profile: cystic fibrosis. November 27, 2002. http://www.ornl.gov/sci/techresources/Human_Genome/posters/chromosome/cf.shtml. Accessed July 2, 2010.

13. Madison, NJ: Quest Diagnostics Incorporated. Human genetics: cystic fibrosis carrier screening: helping you make an informed decision. PP0490. August, 2001. http://www.questdiagnostics.com/healthwise/files/cf.pdf. Accessed July 2, 2010.

14. American Association for Clinical Chemistry. Lab Tests Online Web site. Cystic fibrosis. Modified June 18, 2010. http://labtestsonline.org/understanding/conditions/cystic_fibrosis-6.html#. Accessed July 2, 2010.

15. National Institute of Diabetes and Digestive and Kidney Diseases (NIDDK), National Institutes of Health, U.S. Department of Health and Human Services. Cystic fibrosis research directions: NIDDK. NIH Publication No. 97–4200, July 1997. E-text posted: 12 February 1998. http://www.cureresearch/artic/cystic_fibrosis_research_directions_niddk.htm. Accessed July 2, 2010.

16. McCallum TJ, Milunsky JM, Cunningham DL, Harris DH, Maher TA, Oates RD. Fertility in men with cystic fibrosis: an update on current surgical practices and outcomes. *Chest*. 2000;118:1059-1062.

17. Gilljam M, Antoniou M, Shin J, Dupuis A, Corey M, Tullis DE. Pregnancy in cystic fibrosis: fetal and maternal outcome. *Chest*. 2000;118:85-91.

18. Morral N, Bertranpetit C, Estivill X, et al. The origin of the major cystic fibrosis mutation (delta F508) in European populations. *Nat Genet*. 1994;8:216-218.

19. Romeo G, Devoto M, Galietta LJ. Why is the cystic fibrosis gene so frequent? *Hum Genet*. 1989;84:1-5.

20. Rodman DM, Zamudio S. The cystic fibrosis heterozygote—advantage in surviving cholera? *Med Hypotheses*. 1991;36:253-258.

21. Modiano G, Ciminelli BM, Pignatti PF. Cystic fibrosis and lactase persistence: a possible correlation. *Eur J Hum Genet*. 2007;15:255-259.

22. Centers for Disease Control and Prevention, U.S. Department of Health and Human Services. Reported cases of Lyme disease by year, United States, 1994-2008. http://www.cdc.gov/ncidod/dvbid/lyme/Id_UpClimbLymeDis.htm. Accessed August 20, 2010.

23. Lyme and Tick-Borne Diseases Research Center, Columbia University Medical Center, Scientific Conferences. Lyme & other tick-borne diseases: 34 years, from Lyme, Connecticut across the nation. October 23, 2009; National Harbor, Maryland. http://cait.cpmc.columbia.edu:88/dept/pi/nyspi/LymeDisease/research/scientific.htm. Accessed August 20, 2010.

24. Centers for Disease Control and Prevention, U.S. Department of Health and Human Services. Lyme disease (*borrelia burgdorferi*): 2008 case definition. http://www.cdc.gov/ncphi/disss/nndss/casedef/lyme_disease_2008.htm. Accessed August 20, 2010.

25. Cameron D, Gaito A, Harris N, et al., and the ILADS Working Group. The International Lyme and Associated Diseases Society: evidence-based guidelines for the management of Lyme disease. *Expert Rev. Anti-infect. Ther*. 2004;2:S1-S13.

26. Fallon BA, Keilp JG, Corbera KM, et al. A randomized, placebo-controlled trial of repeated IV antibiotic therapy for Lyme encephalopathy. *Neurology*. 2008;70:992-1003.

27. Rose M. Newsbriefs: origins of syphilis. *Archaeology*. 1997;50:1-2. www.archaeology.org/9701/newsbriefs/syphilis.html. Accessed August 11, 2010.

28. Harper KN, Ocampo PS, Steiner BM, et al. On the origin of the treponematoses: a phylogenetic approach. *PLoS Negl Trop Dis*. 2008;2:e148.

29. Centers for Disease Control and Prevention, U.S. Department of Health and Human Services. Sexually transmitted diseases surveillance, 2008: table 25. primary and secondary syphilis—reported cases and rates by state/area and region listed in alphabetical

order: United States and outlying areas, 2004-2008. http://www.cdc.gov/STD/stats08/tables/25.htm. Accessed August 25, 2010.

30. Centers for Disease Control and Prevention, U.S. Department of Health and Human Services. Sexually transmitted diseases surveillance, 2008: syphilis. http://www.cdc.gov/std/stats08/syphilis.htm. Accessed August 25, 2010.

31. Centers for Disease Control and Prevention, U.S. Department of Health and Human Services. Sexually transmitted diseases surveillance, 2008: STDs in racial and ethnic minorities. http://www.cdc.gov/std/stats08/minorities.htm. Accessed August 25, 2010.

32. Baláž P, Sedlák J. Arsenic in cancer treatment: challenges for application of realgar nanoparticles (a minireview). *Toxins.* 2010;2:1568-1581.

CHAPTER SEVEN
THE DIMENSION OF SIGHT

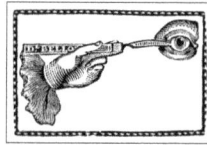

1. de Gelder B, Tamietto M, van Boxtel G, et al. Intact navigation skills after bilateral loss of striate cortex. *Curr Biol.* 2008;18:R1128-R1129.

2. Chaos is a personage who along with Gaia, Tartaros, and Eros emerges from nothing and in turn is able to reproduce parthenogenically. Her two offspring, Erebos (Darkness) and Nyx (Night) mate in order to produce their opposites, Aeither (Brightness) and Hemera (Day). Resuming parthenogenic reproduction, Nyx brings forth a host of entities associated with darkness and conflict. One of these, Eris (Discord) produces fifteen entities representative of specific discords. Each of these, Hardship, Battles, Quarrels, Murders, Forgetfulness, Wars, Lies, Disputes, Starvation, Manslaughters, Ruin, Anarchy, Pains, Oath, and Stories, expresses pathology associated with the dimension of sight.

3. MedlinePlus Web site. U.S. National Library of Medicine, National Institutes of Health. Cluster headache. http://www.nlm.nih.gov/medlineplus/ency/article/000786.htm. Accessed July 25, 2010.

4. Bruehl S. An update on the pathophsiology of complex regional pain syndrome. *Anesthesiol.* 2010;113:713-725.

5. Oaklander AL, Rissmiller JG, Gelman LB, Zheng L, Chang Y, Gott R. Evidence of focal small-fiber axonal degeneration in complex regional pain syndrome-I (reflex sympathetic dystrophy). *Pain.* 2006;120:235-243.

6. National Institute of Neurological Disorders and Stroke Web site. National Institutes of Health. Complex regional pain syndrome fact sheet. http://www.ninds.gov/disorders/reflex_sympathetic_dystrophy/detail_reflex_sympathetic_dystrophy.htm. Accessed July 25, 2010.

7. Marcus H, Adam P, Lennox G, Laing R. Medically unexplained neurological symptoms. *J R Soc Med Sh Rep.* 2010;1:1258-1260.

8. Carson AJ, Ringbauer B, Stone J, McKenzie L, Warlow C, Sharpe M. Do medically unexplained symptoms matter? a prospective cohort study of 300 new referrals to neurology outpatient clinics. *J Neurol Neurosurg Psychiatry.* 2000;68:207-210.

9. Vuilleumier P. Hysterical conversion and brain function. *Prog Brain Res.* 2005;150:309-329.

10. Vuilleumier P, Chicherio C, Assal F, Schwartz S, Slosman D, Landis T. Functional neuroanatomical correlates of hysterical sensorimotor loss. *Hum Mol Genet.* 2001;124(special review issue):1077-1090.

11. Vermeulen F. *Prisma: The Arcana of Materia Medica Illuminated: Similars and Parallels Between Substance and Remedy.* Haarlem, The Netherlands: Emryss b.v. Publishers; 2002.

12. Thurber J. *My Years With Ross.* New York, NY: HarperCollins Publishers Inc.; 2001.

CHAPTER EIGHT

ENCOUNTERING SCYLLA: CONSCIOUSNESS AND CANCER

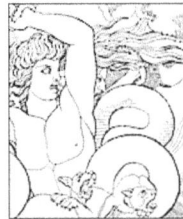

1. Weinberg RA. *One Renegade Cell: The Quest for the Origin of Cancer.* London, England: Weidenfeld & Nicolson; 1998.

2. Louis Klein,, FSHom, a renowned homeopathic teacher and founder and past president of the North American Society of Homeopaths, avers that "failed rebellion" is an important theme within cancer. Klein also relates the theme of failed rebellion generally to bacteria associated with cancer, and links the theme specifically to a group of bacteria, the *Corynebacterium*, with regard to certain cancers. See Klein L. *Miasms and Nosodes: The Origins of Disease, Volume I.* Kandern, Germany: Narayana Publishers GmbH; 2009:133.

3. Further quotes from John Milton's *Paradise Lost, Book I* convey Satan's charisma and hunger to create his own domain:

Thus far these beyond
Compare of mortal prowess, yet observed
Their dread Commander. He, above the rest
In shape and gesture proudly eminent,
Stood like a tower. His form had yet not lost
All her original brightness, nor appeared
Less than Archangel ruined, and th' excess
Of glory obscured

*   *   *   *   *

There went a fame in Heaven that he ere long
Intended to create, and therein plant
A generation whom his choice regard
Should favour equal to the Sons of Heaven.

4. Reich wrote, "German fascism made an all-out effort to anchor itself in the psychic structures of the masses and therefore placed the greatest emphasis upon the inculcation of the adolescents and children. It had no other means at its disposal than the rousing and cultivation of slavery to authority, the basic precondition of which is ascetic, sex-negating education." Reich W. *The Mass Psychology of Fascism*. Carfagno VR, trans. New York, NY: Straus & Giroux; 1970:192.

5. National Cancer Institute, National Institute of Environment Health Sciences, U.S. National Institutes of Health Web site. Cancer and the environment: what you need to know, what you can do. NIH Publication No. 03–2039; August 2003. http:www.cancer.gov/images/Documents/5d17e03e-b39f-4b40-a214-e9e9099c4220/Cancer%20and%20the%20Environment.pdf. Accessed October 10, 2010.

6. National Toxicology Program, Department of Health and Human Services Web site. Report on carcinogens, eleventh edition: introduction. January 31, 2005. http://ntp.nieh.nih.gov//ntp/roc/eleventh/intro.pdf. Accessed October 10, 2010.

7. Sagar J, Chaib B, Sales K, Winslet M, Seifalian A. Role of stem cells in cancer therapy and cancer stem cells: a review. *Cancer Cell Int*. 2007;7:9.

8. Tang C, Ang BT, Pervaiz S. Cancer stem cell: target for anti-cancer therapy. *Faseb J*. 2007;21:3777-3785.

9. Parkin, DM. The global health burden of infection-associated cancers in the year 2002. *Int J Cancer*. 2006;118:3030-3044.

10. National Cancer Institute, U.S. National Institutes of Health Web site. What you need to know about cancer: risk factors. October 4, 2006. http://www.cancer.gov/cancertopics/wyntk/cancer/page4. Accessed October 10, 2010.

11. Zimmer C. Old viruses resurrected through DNA. *New York Times*. November 7, 2006. http://www.nytimes.com/2006/11/07/science/07virus.html. Accessed October 12, 2010.

12. Belyi VA, Levine AJ, Skalka AM. Unexpected inheritance: multiple integrations of ancient Bornavirus and Ebolavirus/Marburgvirus sequences in vertebrate genomes. *PLoS Pathog*. 6(7): e100030. doi:10.1371/journal.ppat.1001030.

13. For other homeopathic cancer treatments, see especially the "Dr. A.U. Ramakrishnan Treatment Protocol," described in the book by Coulter CR and Ramakrishnan AU. *A Homoeopathic Approach to Cancer*. St. Louis, Missouri: Quality Medical Publishing Inc.; 2001.

This work by Dr. Ramakrishnan, a highly respected Indian homeopath who has treated at least five thousand cases of cancer, was long-awaited by members of the homeopathy community. His refinement in treating cancer involves two major modifications of the classical approach: 1) Remedies are chosen, which while not ceasing to address a specific constitutional picture with its own attendant issues of consciousness, also directly target a focal cancer tissue or system; and 2) As opposed to any of several classical, less time-consuming means of administering remedies, Ramakrishnan's method takes longer: For two and a half hours, daily, the patient is obliged to self-administer a highly potentized solution of his or her remedy according to a procedure of adding dilutions for supplemental doses of a remedy known as "plussing."

Other notable homeopaths who have worked extensively with cancer treatment are the late Arthur Hill Grimmer M.D., who pioneered the use of cadmium salts; and, currently, Dr. Prasanta Banerji and Dr. Pratip Banerji of the Prasanta Banerji Homeopathic Research Foundation in Kolkata, India, who appear to have developed an impressive cancer treatment called the "Banerji Protocol."

In my own practice I have found that cancer care options are available for study within acupuncture and homeopathy that are barely known to even seasoned practitioners. I have seen, for example, both benign and malignant tumors shrink after intense acupuncture treatment by scarring moxibustion at one acupuncture point, called Pee Gun (root of tumor). Although many practitioners are reluctant to use scarring moxibustion, my experience with Pee Gun, taught to me by my first acupuncture teacher, James Tin Yau So, is that the practitioner's control of timing and the ability to create distraction during the scarring moxibustion can make the experience endurable for the majority of patients. Immediately following this treatment, the patient often is exhausted, but can feel a powerful sense of well-being.

INDEX

www.ingramcontent.com/pod-product-compliance
Lightning Source LLC
Chambersburg PA
CBHW021554210326
41599CB00010B/439